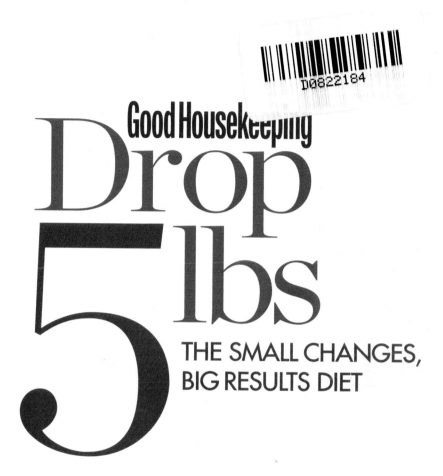

Good Housekeeping

Drop

5 lbs

THE SMALL CHANGES, BIG RESULTS DIET

Good Housekeeping

Drop
5 lbs

THE SMALL CHANGES, BIG RESULTS DIET

Heather K. Jones, RD
Edited by **Rosemary Ellis**, Editor-in-Chief, *Good Housekeeping*

HEARST BOOKS
A division of Sterling Publishing Co., Inc.

New York / London
www.sterlingpublishing.com

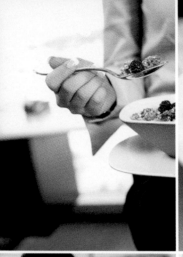
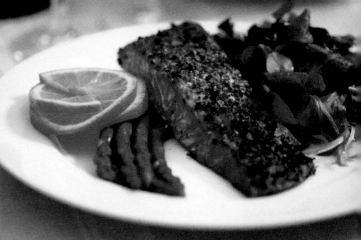
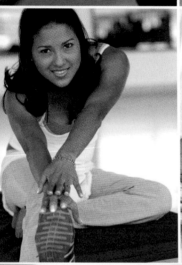
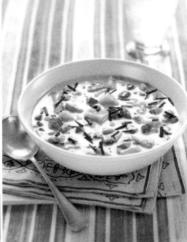
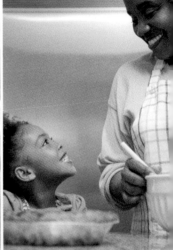
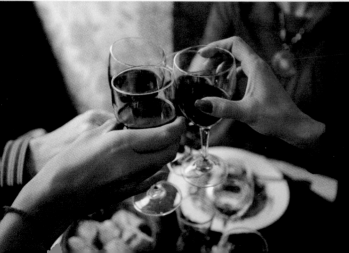
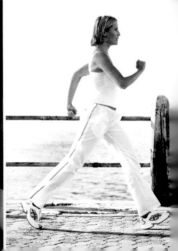

contents

FOREWORD | 6

INTRODUCTION | 8

DIET DECODER QUIZ | 12

THREE-DAY MEAL PLAN | 20

home

CHAPTER 1
Eating In | 26

CHAPTER 2
Supermarket Savvy | 72

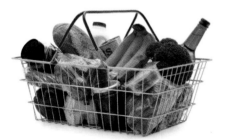

work

CHAPTER 3
On the Job | 108

play

CHAPTER 4
Eating Out | 134

CHAPTER 5
Fitness First | 180

CHAPTER 6
Sweet Celebrations | 208

APPENDIX

DROP 5 CALCULATOR | 246
WORKSHEETS

INDEX TO EATING BEHAVIORS... | 256
AND HOW TO CHANGE THEM

EAT MORE FIBER INDEX | 258

GENERAL INDEX | 259

PHOTOGRAPHY CREDITS | 267

METRIC EQUIVALENT CHARTS | 270

FOREWORD

IT'S NOT HARD TO FIGURE OUT WHY
Good Housekeeping's monthly Drop 5 lbs column is one
of the magazine's most popular features: Most of us,
myself included, want to lose a few pounds at some point.
The Drop 5 column delivers up-to-the-minute, research-
based tips that are easy to follow, fun to read, and proven
to work. So when *Good Housekeeping* decided to produce
a Drop 5 lbs book, we knew it had to be like its namesake.
We put our hands-down best experts on the case: Executive
Editor Jennifer Cook; Nutrition Director Samantha
Cassetty, RD, of the Good Housekeeping Research
Institute; Health Director Toni Hope; Lifestyle Editor
Sara Lyle; and Design Director Courtney Murphy. The
result, which you hold in your hands, is packed with smart
strategies to help you shed weight quickly. And since there's
nothing extreme about the approach—*Good Housekeeping*
is committed to safe, healthy weight loss—you're more
likely to keep the pounds off.

I know—you've tried other diets. The Drop 5 plan is
different from those frustrating one-size-fits-all systems.
The first thing you'll do is figure out your particular diet
downfall by taking our "Diet Decoder Quiz" (page 12).
Then, throughout the chapters, look for custom-tailored
pointers and food choices to help you resist *your* trap,
whether it's mindless munching or skipping meals.

I know you're busy, too. You don't want to waste time
shopping for special diet products, then spend hours
preparing them (or, worse, cooking separate meals for your
family). With the Drop 5 plan, you get to eat regular foods.

We give you complete meals based on easy, prepared items such as a rotisserie chicken from the supermarket. There are also plenty of delicious slimmed-down *Good Housekeeping* recipes, which are triple-tested in our kitchens so you know they will work in yours. And we have rounded up tons of diet-friendly choices from dozens of popular restaurants, like Pizza Hut, Starbucks, and Burger King, so you'll know what is safe to select when you eat out. Most important, you won't get bored. In the Drop 5 magazine column, *Good Housekeeping* features savvy lower-calorie swaps for your favorite dishes, whether you're eating at the mall food court, a holiday buffet table, or your own backyard barbecue. You'll find the same here—only lots more.

The reason you want to lose weight makes no difference. Maybe you want to drop those few pounds that followed you home from vacation. Or maybe you'd like to shed ten to fifteen pounds or fifty . . . or even more. Just follow your personalized Drop 5 plan as long as you want—and you'll keep losing. It's about making small changes to net big results.

So, are you ready to start a new, slimmer chapter in your life? Go on, then—turn the page.

ROSEMARY ELLIS
Editor-in-Chief, *Good Housekeeping*

INTRODUCTION

Drop 5 lbs

FAST—AND FOREVER!

WHETHER YOU'RE TRYING TO SHIMMY back into your skinny jeans, planning to look your best for a family wedding, getting ready for bathing-suit season, or just feeling fed up with carrying around extra weight, we're here to help.

Most people hear the word *diet* and can't help but think sacrifice, guilt, and frustration. They start with lofty goals *(I'll exercise every day and cut out all the junk food)*, but soon learn the hard way that all-or-nothing diets are impossible to live with—even for a few weeks. Fortunately, you don't have to drastically change your life to change your waistline. In fact, experts agree that making small modifications, not radical ones, is the key to dropping pounds. Swap your daily sugary, high-fat coffee drink for a lower-calorie version (page 154), for example, and you'll shave hundreds of calories off your daily tally and lose five pounds in just a month!

Drop 5 lbs will show you how to turn minor lifestyle adjustments into major weight-loss results. You'll begin by pinpointing your personal diet pitfalls with our "Diet Decoder Quiz" (page 12). Whatever your particular challenge, in the chapters that follow, you'll discover hundreds of proven weight-loss strategies from leading experts and studies, tailored to tackle those pitfalls. You'll find out how to identify—and avoid—the hidden calories in foods; you'll discover diet-friendly food swaps, meal ideas, and recipes; you'll learn simple mental tricks to avoid overeating and easy, practical ways to up your exercise, so you can burn more calories.

Want to lose more than five pounds? Just keep using our methods until you reach your weight-loss goal. So, let's say you need to lose around twenty pounds. By setting your horizon at just five pounds at a time, you'll feel a boost in confidence as you reach each short-term objective. Five pounds shed will become ten, and ten will become fifteen . . . Before you know it, you will have attained your twenty-pound goal. The Drop 5 method is an easy-to-live-with, healthy, flexible plan. Bonus: You'll set a great example for your family, shedding pounds and showing the whole gang how to adopt healthy habits to last a lifetime!

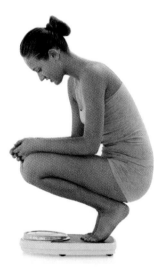

The Science of Weight Loss

Calories. You count them, cut them, obsess about them—but do you know what they actually are? Nutritionally speaking, calories are a measurement of energy. This energy, present in foods and beverages, is burned to keep your body working and moving or else stored as fat for later use. If you consume fewer calories than you burn, you'll lose weight; if you consume more than you burn, you'll gain weight. It's just that simple.

Since one pound of body weight equals about 3,500 calories, to lose that pound you have to either decrease your intake by 3,500 calories or burn 3,500 calories through exercise (or do a combo of cutting calories and upping exercise), over a period of time. If you drop 500 calories a day, for example, you'll lose one pound in a week (500 calories x 7 days = 3,500 calories lost).

If cutting calories leads to weight loss, then drastically cutting calories must lead to very fast weight loss, right? *Wrong.* First, an extreme diet leads to insatiable hunger, priming you for a major diet setback, like a food binge. Even worse, when you don't eat enough calories, you send your body into starvation mode. Your metabolism slows down so your "starving" body can maintain its weight. And that's not all. When you start eating normally again, your metabolism will remain sluggish for a time; that means you will regain weight quickly as your body efficiently stores the suddenly increased calories as fat.

The trick is to create a calorie deficit so you lose weight at a healthy pace—about one to two pounds per week. Our Drop 5 strategies will help you easily shed five pounds in two to three weeks, just in time for that special event. And if your goal is to lose more than five pounds, then the Drop 5 approach to moderate and sustained weight loss can still help you. Here's how it works.

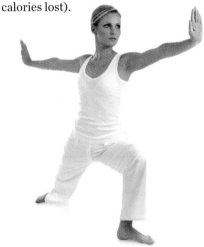

The Drop 5 Way

If you're like most people, you have no idea how much food you consume on a day-to-day basis. Thanks to multitasking, grabbing snacks on the go, scarfing down your kids' leftovers, and various other weight-loss saboteurs, it's hard to keep track of what you eat. Maybe you indulge in more sweets at work because your coworker keeps a candy jar on her desk. Perhaps you have French fries several times a week because you pass McDonald's on the way home. Or maybe every time you worry about money, you retreat to the kitchen for ice cream. But once you begin to notice your patterns, you can figure out ways to change them.

With your diet traps identified, browse the chapters looking for the icons that will help you identify the Drop 5 strategies to try. (Or flip to our "Index to Eating Behaviors . . . and How to Change Them," page 256.) These strategies are designed to shave calories off your daily bottom line and hit the suggested calorie target. For example, eliminate your two-a-day soda habit (page 82), and you can shave off 1,960 calories each week—and drop a pound in under two weeks! While we've already calculated how long it will take you to drop

a pound using each of the selected tips, you can also use the "Drop 5 Calculator Worksheets" in the back of the book (see the examples on pages 19 and 247), plugging in your unique combo of strategies and eating patterns, to determine how long it will take you to lose five pounds.

Remember, your goal is to drop weight at a healthy (and achievable!) rate of about one to two pounds per week. So, while it might seem like a swell idea to combine every tip to try to peel off the pounds in just a few days, if you do, you'll quickly learn it's not only impossible, it's also miserable to even try.

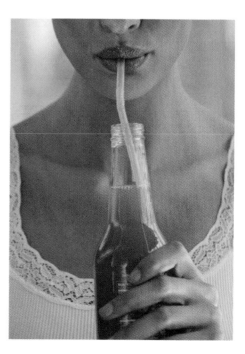

Diet Decoder Quiz

Determine your personal diet pitfalls, and you'll be primed to transform your bad habits into weight-loss success, one small and healthy change at a time. This quick quiz will help you do just that! Circle your answers and tally your results on page 14.

1. **When I'm hungry, fast food is an easy fix; I often stop and grab something—French fries, a burger, maybe a doughnut.**
   A. Rarely (0 points)
   B. Sometimes (1 point)
   C. Often (2 points)
   D. Always (3 points)

2. **While I never think about chips and never buy them, if they're in front of me (at a party or in the office break room, for example), I'll automatically snack on them.**
   A. Rarely (0 points)
   B. Sometimes (1 point)
   C. Often (2 points)
   D. Always (3 points)

3. **I'm usually not hungry in the morning, so I tend to run out of the house without eating breakfast.**
   A. Rarely (0 points)
   B. Sometimes (1 point)
   C. Often (2 points)
   D. Always (3 points)

4. **My hunger is often sudden and urgent, and, if I eat a large quantity of food, I feel guilty afterward.**
   A. Rarely (0 points)
   B. Sometimes (1 point)
   C. Often (2 points)
   D. Always (3 points)

5. **I drink juice, regular soda, or other sugary drinks a few times every day.**
   A. Rarely (0 points)
   B. Sometimes (1 point)
   C. Often (2 points)
   D. Always (3 points)

6. **I drink "sport" or "health" beverages like Gatorade and Vitamin Water.**
   A. Rarely (0 points)
   B. Sometimes (1 point)
   C. Often (2 points)
   D. Always (3 points)

7. **When I am upset, I can eat a whole pizza (or a box of cookies or a carton of ice cream) in one sitting and still want more.**
   A. Rarely (0 points)
   B. Sometimes (1 point)
   C. Often (2 points)
   D. Always (3 points)

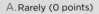

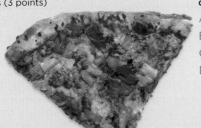

8. **On very busy days, I may eat just one or two times a day.**

   A. Rarely (0 points)

   B. Sometimes (1 point)

   C. Often (2 points)

   D. Always (3 points)

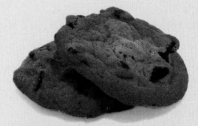

9. **I tend to nibble on whatever foods my family or friends don't finish, even when I'm full.**

   A. Rarely (0 points)

   B. Sometimes (1 point)

   C. Often (2 points)

   D. Always (3 points)

10. **Low-fat pastries and muffins, and sugar-free sweets and cookies are staples in my diet.**

    A. Rarely (0 points)

    B. Sometimes (1 point)

    C. Often (2 points)

    D. Always (3 points)

11. **French fries are my favorite vegetable.**

    A. Rarely (0 points)

    B. Sometimes (1 point)

    C. Often (2 points)

    D. Always (3 points)

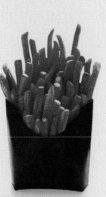

12. **While cooking or preparing food, I'll have so many tastes that I'm not really hungry by the time I sit down to eat the meal.**

    A. Rarely (0 points)

    B. Sometimes (1 point)

    C. Often (2 points)

    D. Always (3 points)

13. **At a certain time of day, I find myself ravenous and searching for something to quiet my growling stomach.**

    A. Rarely (0 points)

    B. Sometimes (1 point)

    C. Often (2 points)

    D. Always (3 points)

14. **After a stressful day, food provides a welcome distraction from my anxious feelings.**

    A. Rarely (0 points)

    B. Sometimes (1 point)

    C. Often (2 points)

    D. Always (3 points)

15. **I hit the drive-thru a few times a week.**

    A. Rarely (0 points)

    B. Sometimes (1 point)

    C. Often (2 points)

    D. Always (3 points)

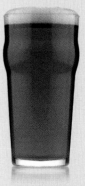

16. **I have at least two beers, glasses of wine, or other alcoholic drinks four or more times a week.**

    A. Rarely (0 points)

    B. Sometimes (1 point)

    C. Often (2 points)

    D. Always (3 points)

17. While watching TV or a movie, I automatically reach for snacks, regardless of whether I'm hungry.

A. Rarely (0 points)

B. Sometimes (1 point)

C. Often (2 points)

D. Always (3 points)

18. Since I'm never sure where and when I'll have a real meal, I tend to eat on the fly.

A. Rarely (0 points)

B. Sometimes (1 point)

C. Often (2 points)

D. Always (3 points)

19. A bad day at work, a fight with a friend, or a family argument can trigger a binge.

A. Rarely (0 points)

B. Sometimes (1 point)

C. Often (2 points)

D. Always (3 points)

20. I have several cups of coffee or tea with sugar and/or cream or milk every day.

A. Rarely (0 points)

B. Sometimes (1 point)

C. Often (2 points)

D. Always (3 points)

TALLY IT UP!

Add points from questions 1, 10, 11, and 15 for your

Junk Food Junkie score: _____ + _____ + _____ + _____ = _____
TOTAL

Add points from questions 2, 9, 12, and 17 for your

Mindless Muncher score: _____ + _____ + _____ + _____ = _____
TOTAL

Add points from questions 3, 8, 13, and 18 for your

Meal Skipper score: _____ + _____ + _____ + _____ = _____
TOTAL

Add points from questions 4, 7, 14, and 19 for your

Emotional Eater score: _____ + _____ + _____ + _____ = _____
TOTAL

Add points from questions 5, 6, 16, and 20 for your

Liquid Calorie Lover score: _____ + _____ + _____ + _____ = _____
TOTAL

THE HIGHEST TOTAL SCORES REPRESENT YOUR PRINCIPAL EATING BEHAVIORS OR HABITS.

You may find that you indulge in more than one (or even all five) of these behaviors. That's okay. If you have a score higher than six on any, just be sure to pay extra attention to the tips targeted to that habit. Throughout the book, the strategies have been tagged to identify the ones that will help you overcome your particular diet pitfalls. For a complete list, see our "Index to Eating Behaviors . . . and How to Change Them," page 256.

 EMOTIONAL EATERS use food for more than fuel—it also serves as a friend and a comfort. Feelings such as sadness, loneliness, anger, or frustration cause these eaters to turn to food for escape.

 JUNK FOOD JUNKIES fill up on nutrient-poor (empty-calorie) foods. Fast foods, sugary snacks, salty munchies, and high-fat fare are the norm; vegetables, fruits, whole grains, and other healthy picks are less frequent choices.

 LIQUID CALORIE LOVERS unwittingly load their diet with extra calories from drinks. Sodas, milkshakes, coffee drinks, cocktails, smoothies, sports drinks, and more spell trouble for their caloric bottom line.

 MEAL SKIPPERS tend to have unbalanced eating patterns and often wait too long between meals. As a result, their meals are not planned or thought out, but rather are last-minute choices made wherever and whenever hunger takes over. They often end up making poor diet choices and caving in on cravings because they're so famished.

 MINDLESS MUNCHERS are all-day grazers and unconscious eaters who put food in their mouths out of habit or boredom, regardless of hunger. They'll eat in front of the TV or automatically snack at a party, for example, paying little attention to their hunger cues. When Mindless Munchers start to track what they consume, they're often surprised at how much they eat during the course of the day.

Remember, transforming just one or two of your daily diet habits can result in pounds lost and a slimmer, trimmer you—in just a few weeks!

Drop 5 Calorie Counts

The Daily Calorie Targets, opposite, provide an easy outline for a diet. While your exact calorie needs depend upon a variety of factors, including your height, weight, and activity levels, for most people, staying within this target will result in a steady rate of weight loss of one to two pounds a week.

For easy reference, we repeat the Daily Calorie Targets at the beginning of each chapter to help guide you as you shop, create healthy meals and snacks at home, and select food from menus.

Think of the total as your daily calorie spending account—if you overdo it at breakfast, just have a lighter lunch. If you have an indulgent snack, cut back a bit at dinner, and so on. As long as you stay within the recommended total calories, you'll still drop pounds.

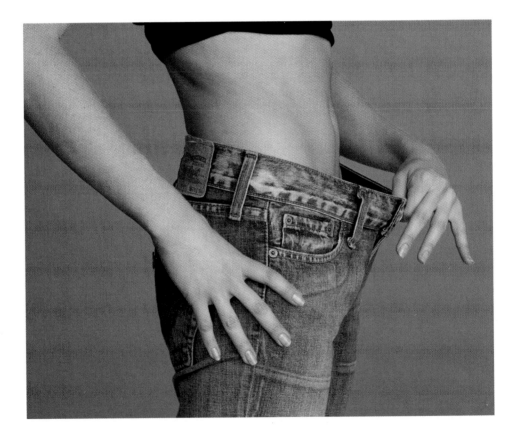

DAILY CALORIE TARGETS

FOR WOMEN		FOR MEN	
Breakfast	350	Breakfast	450
Lunch	500	Lunch	600
Dinner	500	Dinner	600
Snack	100	Snack	200
Optional Treat	100	Optional Treat	200
TOTAL	1,450–1,550	TOTAL	1,850–2,050

Men have more lean tissue (muscle) than women, so they need more calories each day. The Drop 5 meals in this book fall within the calorie guidelines for women. Men will need to add around 100 calories to each meal or snack, either by eating larger portions or by rounding out meals with nutrient-dense foods. Here are some easy ways to add 100 calories to any recipe or meal.

PRODUCE

1 medium sweet potato

1 medium ear of corn

1 large artichoke

1 cup grapes

2 cups cubed melon

1 banana

1 apple

GRAINS

1 slice whole-grain bread

1 whole-wheat English muffin

1 cup whole-grain cereal

¾ cup cooked oats

½ cup cooked brown rice

½ cup cooked whole-wheat couscous

½ cup cooked whole-grain pasta

PROTEIN

1 cup nonfat milk or unsweetened soymilk

1 ounce part-skim string cheese

1 tablespoon peanut butter or 2 tablespoons nuts

½ cup beans

3 ounces broiled or grilled fish

3 ounces broiled or grilled skinless chicken breast

3-ounce can of tuna in water

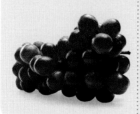

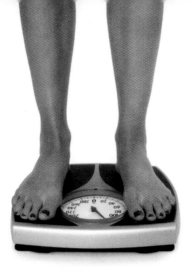

To keep your energy level up and to feel your best, fuel your body with nutrient-packed calories from foods like fruits, veggies, lean proteins, low-fat dairy, whole-grain breads and cereals, and judicious amounts of healthy fats like avocado, olive oil, and canola oil (see "Make the Most of Your Calories," page 22). Have the optional 100-calorie treat once a day, or save up those calories for a larger treat every other day, or enjoy 350-calorie treats a couple of days a week. If you want to cut calories a bit more, you can skip the optional treat altogether.

The delicious and easy-to-prepare meals in this book fall within the Drop 5 calorie targets and are crammed with nutrition. You'll find lots of helpful Drop 5 recipes and recipe makeovers in Chapter 1: Eating In (page 26) and Chapter 6: Sweet Celebrations (page 208). In Chapter 6, you'll also discover ways to avoid holiday weight gain, which, under the Drop 5 plan, no longer has to be inevitable. Our healthy holiday makeover recipes will save you hundreds of calories—Light and Creamy Eggnog (page 229), for example, shaves off more than 300 calories per serving. Or munch on our Light Latkes (page 226); they're 150 calories slimmer than regular ones. In Chapter 2: Supermarket Savvy (page 72), you'll learn how to fill your cart with diet-friendly foods, and in Chapter 3: On the Job (page 108), you'll find easy ways to lose while you work. In Chapter 4: Eating Out (page 134), you'll find plenty of Drop 5 meal options that make losing weight, even while dining out and hitting the drive-thru, a tasty possibility. And in Chapter 5: Fitness First (page 180), you'll learn how exercise can help you lose even faster. Also be sure to check out our sample "Three-Day Meal Plan" on page 20.

Using the Drop 5 Calculator

DROP 5 STRATEGY	CALORIES SAVED OR BURNED	REPETITIONS PER WEEK	TOTAL DROP IN CALORIES
Choose an open-faced sandwich (page 49)	100	5	500
Swap a coffeehouse mocha for a home-made low-fat latte (page 42)	300	5	1,500
Take a yoga class (page 203)	200	2	400
TOTAL CALORIES SAVED OR BURNED PER WEEK			2,400

Our Drop 5 Calculator makes it easy to track your daily and weekly drop in calories so you can achieve your weight-loss goals. Here is how it works.

Our sample dieter has chosen three diet strategies. She's having her lunch sandwich open-faced, eliminating five slices of bread a week; she's given up her weekday mocha coffee habit for a less caloric latte; and she's started taking a yoga class twice a week. Above, she's noted the calories she's saved or burned to calculate her total drop in calories.

HOW LONG WILL IT TAKE THIS DIETER TO DROP 5? Simply divide the drop in calories required to lose one pound **(3,500)** by her actual drop in calories in a week **(2,400)** and you'll get the time it will take her to lose **1 pound:**

$$3,500 \div 2,400 = 1.46 \text{ WEEKS}$$

Multiply by 5 to find out how long it will take her to lose **5 pounds:**

$$1.46 \times 5 = 7.3 \text{ WEEKS}$$

HOW LONG WILL IT TAKE *YOU* TO LOSE WEIGHT? Just insert your personal diet strategies into the worksheets we've provided on page 248. Do some simple math, and—voilà!—you'll find out how long it will take you to Drop 5.

Three-Day Meal Plan

Combine any of the Drop 5 breakfasts, lunches, dinners, snacks, and treats in this book, or create your own Drop 5 meals that stay within the Daily Calorie Targets (page 17), and you'll lose about one to two pounds each week.

Here are three sample days' worth of meals to get you started. We've designed this mini plan to be simple and quick, with eat-out and eat-in options, so you can see how smart choices add up to weight loss. Whenever a meal is over (or under) the calorie limit, we've compensated with a

lower (or higher) calorie total for the meal. You can do the same as you devise your own plan. Use this one here for ideas on how to mix and match the Drop 5 recipes and meals coming up. In addition to all the food and drinks listed in the meal plan, you can have as many calorie-free beverages (water, tea, coffee, sugar-free sodas, seltzer) as you like, as well as sugar substitutes including Splenda, Equal, NutraSweet, and stevia. You can also fill your plate with lots of low-calorie vegetables (see page 89).

DAY ONE

Breakfast Apple Pie Oatmeal (page 42) served with 14 whole almonds on the side and coffee or tea **321 CALORIES**

Lunch Subway Sweet Onion Chicken Teriyaki Sub with 1 Dannon Light & Fit Yogurt (any flavor) **460 CALORIES**

Snack Fruit and Cheese: ½ pear, sliced and topped with 1 tablespoon crumbled blue cheese **120 CALORIES**

Dinner Salmon and Black Bean Tortilla Salad (page 79) **514 CALORIES**

Treat 1 mango, sliced **135 CALORIES**

TOTAL DAY ONE 1,550 CALORIES

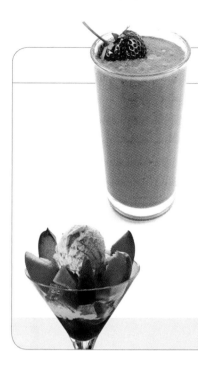

DAY TWO

Breakfast Strawberry Mania Smoothie
(page 155) **326 CALORIES**

Lunch Kashi Pocket Bread Chicken Rustico
Sandwich served with ½ cup grapes and 1 part-
skim mozzarella stick **458 CALORIES**

Snack 2 tablespoons hummus with ½ small red
pepper, sliced, for dipping **125 CALORIES**

Dinner Pizza and Salad: 2 slices medium
(12-inch) Thin 'N Crispy Crust Veggie Lover's
Pizza Hut pizza paired with 2 cups mixed greens
tossed with 10 pumps spray dressing and, for
dessert, 1 cup mixed berries **453 CALORIES**

Treat Peaches and Cream (page 68)
133 CALORIES

TOTAL DAY TWO **1,495** CALORIES

DAY THREE

Breakfast Blueberry Muffin (page 39) paired
with 1 orange and a quickie latte (2 to 3
tablespoons powdered espresso mixed with
1 cup fat-free milk and heated in microwave for
1 minute) **327 CALORIES**

Lunch Simple Sandwich (page 116) served with
around 100 calories prepared soup, such as
Campbell's Soup at Hand Vegetable with Mini
Round Noodles. **505 CALORIES**

Snack Starbucks Tall Skinny Caramel Latte
90 CALORIES

Dinner Spinach and Tortellini (page 90)
served with 2 cups mixed greens and tossed with
10 to 15 pumps spray vinaigrette **460 CALORIES**

Treat Whole Treat Organic Fudge Bar
100 CALORIES

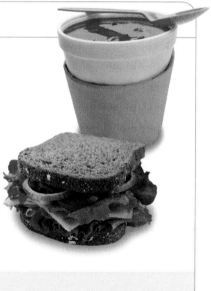

TOTAL DAY THREE **1,482** CALORIES

Drop 5 Strategies for Weight Loss

To get you started, here are our top tips for slimming down—and keeping the pounds off. Make these strategies your mantra, and you will drop that weight. Tape them up on your wall, computer, dashboard—wherever you'll see them—to keep you motivated.

1 BELIEVE YOU CAN DO IT You've already taken the first step by picking up this book. But if your dieting will wavers along the way, don't give up on yourself. Think about what you're most committed to in life—your family, spouse, faith, a job? Now place yourself and your weight-loss goals and health at the top of that list. And don't forget to acknowledge your successes, no matter how small. You avoided that candy bar staring you down from the vending machine today? Worth a secret inner high five at least! Dropped your first three pounds? Surely justification for that new belt you've had your eye on. For regular pick-me-ups, check out the inspiring Learn from the "Losers" quotes about real diet successes sprinkled throughout the book.

2 MAKE THE MOST OF YOUR CALORIES By selecting empty-calorie foods, you're spending a lot for something that offers very little—like the insanely expensive, very cute shoes that give you blisters and are difficult to walk in. They might be fun to wear on occasion, but most of the time, you'll want to wear something stylish *and* comfortable. If you're economizing on calories to lose weight, it makes sense to pack a lot of nutrition into what you eat. A food that's value-loaded with vitamins, minerals, and fiber, but also low in calories is a nutritional bargain—it's a *nutrient*-dense food. On the other hand, foods like soda and sweets will set you back lots of calories but are low in vitamins and minerals, making them low-nutrient, or *calorie*-dense, foods. Although they are often called empty-calorie foods, empty of nutrients is more like it.

This doesn't mean fries, burgers, sweets, and other less-stellar choices are diet no-no's. The truth is, no food or drink is so high in calories, fat, or sugar that including it *on occasion* in an overall healthful diet is going to keep you from losing weight. Just be sure to keep your total calorie intake within the recommended limits (page 17), and you'll still Drop 5.

HERE'S WHAT TO LOOK FOR:

- **Fruits and vegetables** Rich in nutrients and low in calories, produce is one of a dieter's best friends. There's no such thing as a bad fruit or veggie, but the more variety, the better (page 88).

- **Low-fat dairy** These versions of milk, cheese, yogurt, cottage cheese, and more are packed with nutrition, not calories (page 102).

- **Lean proteins** Grilled or broiled lean meat, poultry, and fish, as well as vegetarian choices like beans and tofu, will help you feel fuller and stay that way (page 96).

- **Whole grains** Select fiber-rich, whole-grain foods like oatmeal, whole-wheat bread, and brown rice instead of refined grains like white bread, white pasta, and white rice (page 84).

- **Healthy fats** Choose olive and canola oils, avocados, nuts and nut butters, seeds, and olives—but remember, a little goes a long, long way. A splash of olive oil in your salad, a small handful of nuts with your cereal, or a few slices of avocado on your sandwich all add satiety and flavor.

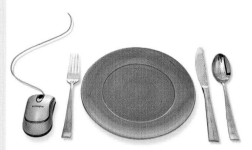

3 GET THE FACTS Be your own food detective, online and off, and you'll not only uncover surprises about what's hiding in your food, you'll also set yourself up for success. Check out Supermarket Savvy (page 72) for easy tips on how to fill your cart with the right foods and Eating Out (page 134) for the insider info you need to make the best choices, no matter where you dine. Start to read food labels (see "Label Lesson," page 24), gather nutrition brochures from your favorite dining spots, and go online to restaurant and food manufacturers' websites to investigate. Also check out this free online calorie counter for basic foods like nuts, cheese, and fruits: www.nal.usda.gov/fnic/foodcomp/search. While there are lots of calorie calculators on the web, this tool from the USDA provides trusted, well-researched information.

LABEL LESSON

Once you get the inside scoop and realize you may be consuming a lot more than you think, you'll be in a better position to make informed decisions about your diet. Take a look at this mac 'n' cheese label to learn how to make the best picks:

Nutrition Facts on packaged food and drink labels are like road-maps to your healthier (and slimmer!) destination.

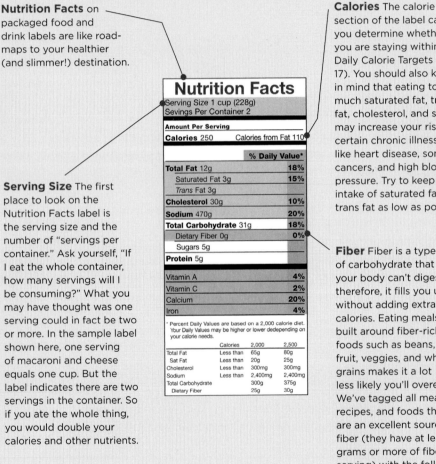

Nutrition Facts

Serving Size 1 cup (228g)
Sevings Per Container 2

Amount Per Serving

Calories 250   Calories from Fat 110

	% Daily Value*
Total Fat 12g	**18%**
Saturated Fat 3g	**15%**
Trans Fat 3g	
Cholesterol 30g	**10%**
Sodium 470g	**20%**
Total Carbohydrate 31g	**18%**
Dietary Fiber 0g	**0%**
Sugars 5g	
Protein 5g	

Vitamin A	**4%**
Vitamin C	**2%**
Calcium	**20%**
Iron	**4%**

* Percent Daily Values are based on a 2,000 calorie diet. Your Daily Values may be higher or lower dedepending on your calorie needs.

		Calories	2,000	2,500
Total Fat	Less than		65g	80g
Sat Fat	Less than		20g	25g
Cholesterol	Less than		300mg	300mg
Sodium	Less than		2,400mg	2,400mg
Total Carbohydrate			300g	375g
Dietary Fiber			25g	30g

Serving Size The first place to look on the Nutrition Facts label is the serving size and the number of "servings per container." Ask yourself, "If I eat the whole container, how many servings will I be consuming?" What you may have thought was one serving could in fact be two or more. In the sample label shown here, one serving of macaroni and cheese equals one cup. But the label indicates there are two servings in the container. So if you ate the whole thing, you would double your calories and other nutrients.

Calories The calorie section of the label can help you determine whether you are staying within the Daily Calorie Targets (page 17). You should also keep in mind that eating too much saturated fat, trans fat, cholesterol, and sodium may increase your risk of certain chronic illnesses like heart disease, some cancers, and high blood pressure. Try to keep your intake of saturated fat and trans fat as low as possible.

Fiber Fiber is a type of carbohydrate that your body can't digest; therefore, it fills you up without adding extra calories. Eating meals built around fiber-rich foods such as beans, fruit, veggies, and whole grains makes it a lot less likely you'll overeat. We've tagged all meals, recipes, and foods that are an excellent source of fiber (they have at least 5 grams or more of fiber per serving) with the following icon to help you find fiber-rich foods fast. For a complete list, see our "Eat More Fiber Index," page 258.

Source: Adapted from the U.S. Food and Drug Administration

4 START MOVING Fred and Ginger, peanut butter and jelly, Romeo and Juliet: These pairs are all better together than apart. The same goes for diet and exercise. Multiple studies show that weight-loss efforts are vastly more successful when dieters reduce calories *and* increase physical activity. The secret is to find things you enjoy so you'll want to keep doing them. And don't forget, everyday activities like gardening and taking the stairs burn calories too. See Fitness First (page 180) for lots of ideas on how to incorporate more movement into your daily routine.

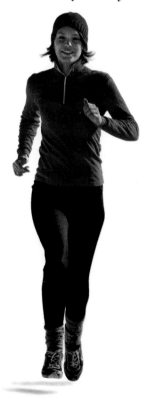

5 CHANGE FOR GOOD *Drop 5 lbs* is designed to reveal your diet traps so you can change your habits and (finally) shake those extra pounds. However, if you don't modify your habits for good, you won't be able to solve your weight problems in the long term. As soon as your old eating habits return, so will the weight. Think about adopting the Drop 5 strategies you learn here permanently. These behaviors, when they become lifelong practices, will help you achieve and maintain your ultimate goal— whether it's weight loss or healthier living.

Once you hit your desired weight, add around 100 calories to your daily intake. After a week, weigh yourself at your usual time, on your usual scale. If you have lost any weight, add another 100 calories to your daily total. Repeat until your weight remains stable—that's how much you need each day to stop losing weight and sustain the weight loss you've accomplished.

So give it a try. Read on to learn how to overcome your personal weight-loss hurdles—whether those are junk food cravings, bad exercise habits, skipping meals, emotional eating, or some combination of these or others. Once you do, you'll find that you will Drop 5 in no time!

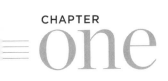
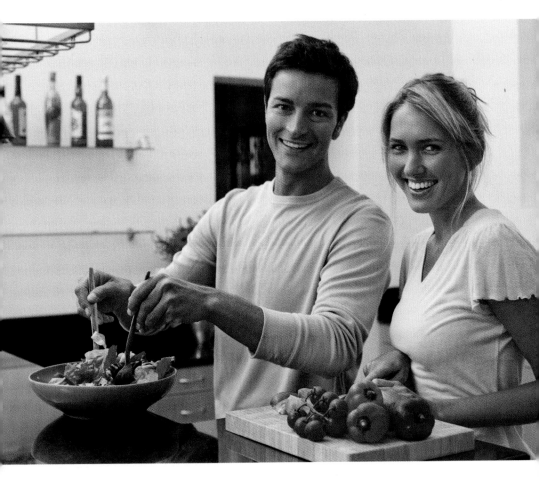

EATING IN
cooking for
weight
loss

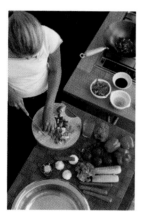

Our healthy recipes and home-cooking tips and tricks will inspire you to eat healthier and drop pounds.

I F YOU WANT TO HAVE A HEALTHIER DIET, enjoy delicious and satisfying meals, and finally win the war against unwanted pounds, eating at home is a key strategy. Dining in gives you the most control over your diet. It also allows you to avoid the tempting bread baskets, fat-laden dishes, and calorie-dense desserts that you find in restaurants. Plus, as restaurant servings keep getting bigger, so do pants sizes!

Food is one of life's great pleasures—especially preparing and sharing it with family and friends—and eating in provides you full command over your choices and portions. You can also experiment with new ingredients and taste good-for-your-waistline recipes and foods. This chapter has been designed to help you Drop 5 with meals so tasty you won't miss the extra calories and fat. With an abundance of tips and advice accompanying the delicious and easy-to-prepare recipes, this is your guide to practicing good, at-home eating habits.

Dining well at home doesn't have to be about following a strict set of rules or giving up your favorite foods. Instead, it's about making commonsense choices. Turn the page for the Drop 5 Top 5 tips to help make your home a weight-loss-friendly environment every day.

Drop Top 5

5 EATING IN HOW-TOS

1 **DETOX YOUR KITCHEN** Clear your cupboards, fridge, and freezer of the foods you know will get you in trouble, and instead stock up on healthy and tasty options you and your family will enjoy. Conduct your own in-house taste tests—ask your family to get involved, try new lower-calorie recipes and new foods, and gain a new (and healthy!) weight-loss perspective. (See "Kitchen Cleanup" on page 34 to find out what to toss and what to keep.)

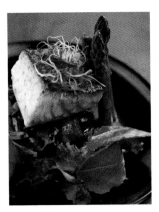

Substitute ingredients used in everyday cooking with healthier options (like this grilled halibut) and you'll slash calories for Drop 5 success.

2 **MAKE IT OVER** Substitute ingredients used in everyday cooking with healthier options and you'll slash calories—and propel yourself to Drop 5 success. The cooking tricks you'll learn will not only help you maintain your desired weight once you get there, you'll also pass this useful knowledge on to your family.

Here are some tips for trimming excess fat and calories from your home-cooked meals:

- Choose lean cuts of meat (page 97) and trim all visible fat before cooking. Remove skin from poultry before or after cooking.

- Broil meat on a rack so the fat can drip away and be discarded.

- Use at least 92 percent lean ground beef, or substitute ground chicken or turkey for ground beef. Be sure the package is labeled "meat only," or the poultry versions may contain skin and therefore have as much fat as ground beef.

- Look for fish canned in water (not oil). Or, for an even easier packaged fish, pick up no-fuss vacuum-packed pouches of tuna and salmon to toss into salads, sandwiches, or your favorite recipes.

- Choose low-cal fish and shellfish, and use a healthy cooking method such as baking, broiling, roasting, braising, grilling, or stir-frying.

- Eliminate all or some of the grated cheese in recipes; instead, sprinkle a small amount over already cooked dishes to maximize the taste.

- Substitute protein-packed canned legumes like beans and lentils for meat in casseroles; the dish will have fewer calories and more filling fiber.

- Prepare soups and stews ahead of time and chill them overnight so you can remove all the hardened fat from the surface.

- Be skimpy with fat. Use nonstick pans or nonstick cooking spray with your regular pans.

- Experiment with nonfat flavorings—squeeze orange or lemon juice into stews or over meats; add citrus zest, soy sauce, fresh ginger, hot peppers, herbs, or tomato sauce to your favorite recipes.

- Spritz olive oil spray on fish or chicken before seasoning and broiling them to minimize fat and maximize the taste of herbs and spices. Spray oil on vegetables (rather than brushing it on) to cut down on fat.

- Choose low-fat and nonfat milk, reduced fat and low-fat sour cream and cheese, and nonfat yogurt for recipes. They provide the same amounts of calcium and protein as whole-milk varieties.

- Reduce the amount of nuts in cookies, brownies, cakes, and breads to just a few tablespoons for fewer calories.

- For an index to the healthy recipes in this book, see page 32.

Decide to dine in: Restaurant meals have a lot more calories (at least 60 percent more, according to one recent study) than the same dishes prepared at home.

3 DOWNSIZE YOUR DISHES Use smaller plates, bowls, and glasses for everyday meals.

According to a Cornell University study, people tend to serve themselves 30 percent more food when given large bowls and spoons. And research at the Food and Brand Lab at the University of Illinois found that people who used short, wide glasses poured 76 percent more soda, milk, or juice than when they used tall, slender ones.

No need to buy new; simply swap your dinner plate for a salad plate, a soup bowl for a mug, or a regular glass for a juice glass. Or, if you have oversized dishes and glasses, use measuring cups to familiarize yourself with calorie-controlled portions and keep these studies in mind as you ladle out servings.

DAILY CALORIE TARGETS

Consult these guidelines as you choose recipes, meals, and snacks from this chapter.

FOR WOMEN		FOR MEN	
Breakfast	350	Breakfast	450
Lunch	500	Lunch	600
Dinner	500	Dinner	600
Snack	100	Snack	200
Optional Treat	100	Optional Treat	200
TOTAL	1,450–1,550	Total	1,850–2,050

If you go a little over (or under) at any meal, compensate by adjusting your calories later in the day. Have the optional treat once a day, or save up those calories and have a larger treat every other day, or even two larger 350-calorie treats a couple of days a week. If you want to cut calories a bit more, you can also skip the optional treat altogether.

4 **CONTROL CRAVINGS** Whether it's chocolate or chips, ice cream or whipped cream, the foods people crave have one thing in common: They are calorie-dense, a Tufts University study recently confirmed. But in that study, the researchers also noted that while virtually everyone has cravings, the dieters in the group who successfully lost weight or kept it off gave in to their must-haves—just less often.

Instead of denying your craving and later binging on that favorite food, "accept that cravings are normal, and then deal with them," advises Susan Roberts, PhD, professor of nutrition and psychiatry at Tufts. "Sometimes you can give in, and sometimes you need to brush your teeth and wait for the desire to pass." (For even more help dealing with at-home emotional eating, see page 71.)

5 **PAY ATTENTION** A recent study showed that Americans use external cues, like waiting till their TV show is over, to stop eating, unlike the don't-get-fat French, who rely on internal messages, such as feeling full. We're also susceptible to social influences. "Many of us keep eating until almost everyone at the table is finished," says Brian Wansink, PhD, a nutrition expert at Cornell University and the author of *Mindless Eating*. If you tend to finish before your family, he suggests, "keep the salad bowl or veggies in front of you," rather than picking at the macaroni and cheese. Better yet, ask yourself if you're really still hungry. Unless the answer is truly yes, put down your fork.

BE SURE TO CHECK OUT OUR HEALTHY RECIPES

In addition to these mealtime recipes, you'll find dozens of suggestions for easy-to-prepare, good-for-you snacks and treats sprinkled throughout this book. See also our "Eat More Fiber Index" on page 258.

(Note: Yellow highlights indicate foods shown in photographs.)

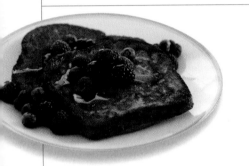

BREAKFAST
- Black Bean and Salsa Omelet, page 40
- Blueberry Muffins, page 39
- Broccoli-Cheddar Scramble, page 92
- French Toast, page 43
- Garden Vegetable Omelet, page 40
- Western-Style Omelet, page 41
- Red Pepper and Goat Cheese Omelet, page 41
- Spinach, Cheese, and Bacon Omelet, page 41
- Spinach Scramble, page 90
- Strawberry Mania, page 155

APPETIZERS AND DRINKS
- Black Bean Dip, page 50
- Guiltless Guacamole, page 167
- Homemade Café au Lait, page 42
- Light and Creamy Eggnog, page 229
- Sour Cream and Onion Party Dip, page 242

SOUPS, SANDWICHES, AND SALADS
- Black Bean Soup, page 51
- Caribbean Wrap, page 98
- Chicken and Rice Salad, page 45
- Corn and Chicken Pasta Salad, page 92
- Dijon Bean and Veggie Salad, page 45
- Greek Steak Salad, page 101
- Greek Chicken Burgers, page 173
- Honey Mustard Chicken Salad, page 45
- Kidney Bean Chili, page 51
- Lime Tuna and Black Bean Salad, page 45
- New England Clam Chowder, page 66
- Open-Faced Chicken Quesadilla, page 98
- Open-Faced Mexican Veggie Burrito, page 92
- Salmon and Black Bean Tortilla Salad, page 79
- Spinach and Hummus Flatbread, page 90
- Spinach Salad with Chicken, page 90
- Sweet and Savory Salmon Salad, page 45
- Tuna English Muffins, page 79
- Tuna Salad, page 48
- Tuscan Tuna Salad, page 79
- Waldorf Salad, page 98

MAIN DISHES
- Chicken and Artichoke Pasta, page 98
- Chicken Breasts Provençal, page 63

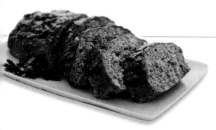

- Chicken Breasts with Apple-Curry Sauce, page 62
- Chicken Breasts with Black Bean Salsa, page 63
- Chicken Breasts with Chinese Ginger Sauce, page 63
- Chicken Breasts with Dijon Sauce, page 62
- Confetti Pasta, page 58
- Creamy Mushroom Cavatappi, page 175
- Mediterranean Couscous, page 98
- Meat Loaf, page 57
- Orange-Fennel Pasta, page 58
- Pasta with Peas and Onion, page 59
- Pasta with Tomatoes and Lemon, page 59
- Pasta with Tuna Puttanesca, page 79
- Marinara Pasta, page 59
- Red-Cooked Chicken with Assorted Vegetables, page 61
- Roasted Salmon with Squash, page 65
- Salmon Cakes, page 79
- Sesame Shrimp and Asparagus Stir-Fry, page 169
- Shepherd's Pie, page 67
- Shrimp Rice with Baby Peas, page 92
- Snow Pea Stir-Fry, page 98
- Spinach and Tortellini, page 90
- Spinach and White Bean Pasta, page 90
- Steak Fajita Wraps, page 101
- Steak Fried Rice, page 101
- Steak Pesto Pasta, page 101
- Thai Steak Noodles, page 101
- Turkey Fajitas, page 171
- Whole-Wheat Penne Genovese, page 177

SIDE DISHES

- Black-Eyed Pea Sauté, page 221
- Garbanzo Bean Salad, page 226
- Holiday Herb-Roasted Potatoes, page 236
- Lean Green Bean Casserole, page 98
- Light Latkes, page 226
- Potato Salad, page 236
- Vegetable-Herb Stuffing, page 223

DESSERTS

- Angel Food Cake, page 241
- Balsamic Berries, page 68
- Better Banana Pudding, page 237
- Chocolate Chip Cookies, page 70
- Chocolate Figs, page 68
- Coffee Granita, page 68
- Lighter Brownies, page 233
- Peaches and Cream, page 68
- PB Pudding, page 68
- Poached Pears with Fresh Ginger, page 224
- Pumpkin Spice Ring, page 224
- Strawberry Ice Cream, page 69

KITCHEN
cleanup

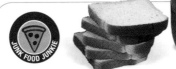

Here's a list of items to purge from your kitchen—and, following that, our favorite must-haves to stock up on. Donate unopened foods to a local soup kitchen, or use up what you have on hand, then replace with our picks.

Purge Your Pantry

Toss out high-calorie, nutrient-poor foods including:

- Chips
- Candy
- White-flour snacks (like crackers and pretzels)
- Cookies
- Sugary cereal
- Pastries
- Cakes
- White bread
- Cream-based foods (like chowders, soups, creamed vegetables)
- Vegetable shortening
- Cheese sauce and fatty dips
- Creamy salad dressing

- Full-fat mayo
- Full-fat dairy products
- Full-fat ground beef (lean ground beef— 92 percent or higher— is okay)
- Meat sausages
- Canned meats
- Full-fat beef hot dogs (reduced-fat hot dogs are okay— see page 235)
- Regular soda (diet soda is okay)
- Sweetened teas
- Juice drinks

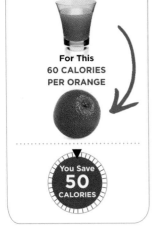

SIMPLE SWAPS

Swap This
110 CALORIES
PER 8-OUNCE
SERVING
ORANGE JUICE

For This
60 CALORIES
PER ORANGE

You Save
50
CALORIES

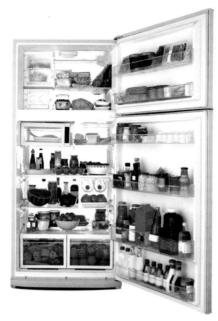

Learn from the "Losers"

"I discovered that there are two types of hunger. One is real hunger in the pit of your stomach; the other is any empty feeling you think is hunger—and it's something food can't fill. Now I treat my body like a car and only give it fuel when it is close to empty."

—HEATHER SANCHEZ,
85 POUNDS LOST

MUST-HAVES FOR YOUR REFRIGERATOR

Add these fridge essentials to your weekly shopping list so that they are always on hand.

1. Seasonal fresh fruit and vegetables (page 88)

2. Cheese—low-fat sliced, shredded, or string cheese, or small amounts of strong cheeses like blue, feta, or Parmesan for a lower-calorie flavor lift (page 102)

3. Hummus—plain or flavored

4. Low-fat or nonfat milk (or soy milk), cottage cheese, and yogurt (page 103)

5. Eggs or egg substitute (for more on cholesterol and eggs, see page 104)

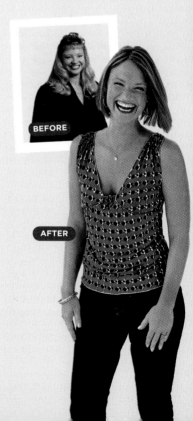

BEFORE

AFTER

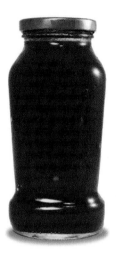

MUST-HAVES FOR YOUR PANTRY

Once you've cleaned out the shelves, it's time to fill them with healthy options.

1. Whole grains such as wheat berries and whole-wheat couscous, barley, and pasta (see our Drop 5 whole-grain pasta meal ideas on page 58 and "Healthy Convenience Grain Dishes" on page 85)

2. Jarred low-fat sauces such as marinara, salsa, soy sauce, etc.

3. Whole-wheat breads, wraps, rolls, pitas, tortillas, etc. (page 87)

4. Canned beans (see page 50 for recipes), salmon and tuna (in water, not oil), low-fat soups, and fruit in juice or water (no added sugar or syrup)

5. Calorie-controlled portions of snacks, nuts, and treats (pages 54 and 121)

SIMPLE SWAPS

Swap This
140 CALORIES PER
12-OUNCE CAN
REGULAR SODA

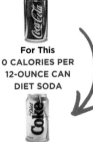

For This
0 CALORIES PER
12-OUNCE CAN
DIET SODA

You Save
140
CALORIES

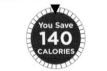

MUST-HAVE CONDIMENTS

Add low-calorie flavor with these extras.

1. Mustard (stone ground, Dijon, etc.)

2. Spray salad dressings

3. Vinegar (balsamic, sherry, red wine, white wine, etc.)

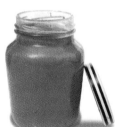

4. Oils (good picks include olive, canola, safflower, flaxseed, and grapeseed oils)

5. Herbs and spices, fresh and dried

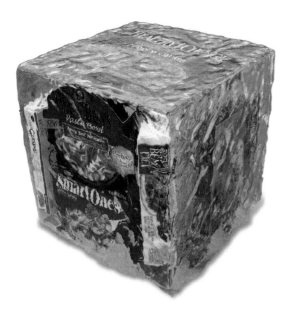

MUST-HAVES FOR YOUR FREEZER

A quick, healthy meal or treat is always just minutes away.

1. Healthy frozen dinners to suit every taste, from Italian to Indian, and plenty of choices in between (see our favorite selections on page 105)

2. Boneless, skinless chicken breasts and fish fillets are easy everyday dinner solutions when paired with a quick sauce (page 62)

3. Packages of frozen fruits and vegetables, with no added sugar, salt, or sauce (see page 92 for recipe ideas)

4. Portions of homemade, low-fat soups and casseroles (see page 67 for our Healthy Recipe Makeover for Shepherd's Pie and page 66 for our lighter New England Clam Chowder)

5. Fruit pops made with real fruit (no added sugar) and other low-cal frozen treats (see our top picks on page 106)

Learn from the "Losers"

"I shop the walls of the grocery store—it's where I find the produce and protein and food that's low in carbohydrates."

—MARY JANE MEDLOCK,
162 POUNDS LOST

"When I'm cooking, I splash Tabasco sauce on everything—the spicy kick makes me eat slower, so I don't consume as much. Another trick: If I have time on the weekend, I'll grill up six chicken breasts, steam some veggies, portion everything into containers, and pop the food into the freezer. Then on weeknights, when I come home from work hungry, I can have a healthy dinner in minutes."

—SHELLEY NAPIER,
206 POUNDS LOST

RETHINK
breakfast

It's no secret that it's the most important meal of the day. In fact, research shows that breakfast eaters typically consume about 100 fewer calories during the course of the day (that's ten pounds a year!) and weigh less than those who forgo food in the morning. Here's how to make it fit into your schedule—and how eating the right breakfast can help you Drop 5.

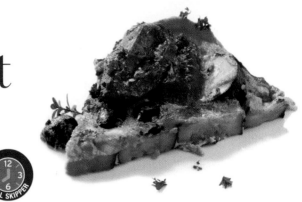

Breakfast Breakdown

These healthy ways to start your day are ready in under ten minutes and tally up to roughly 350 calories each.

- **PITA SPREAD** Toast ½ mini whole-wheat pita. Top with ⅓ cup part-skim ricotta cheese and 1½ tablespoons chopped nuts. Drizzle with 1 teaspoon honey. Serve with 15 red grapes.

- **HOT CEREAL WITH FRUIT** Combine a 2-ounce, prepared single-serving cup instant hot oatmeal with 1 tablespoon dried cranberries, raisins, strawberries, or blueberries. Serve with 1 apple, sliced.

- **ALMOST BAGEL** Top 5 nonfat bagel chips with 2 tablespoons shredded reduced-fat cheese. Microwave 30 seconds or until cheese melts. Serve with 4 ounces orange juice.

- **FRITTATA** Reheat ½ cup leftover veggies, such as sliced zucchini, peppers, or mushrooms, in nonstick skillet coated with cooking spray. Beat 2 eggs with 1 tablespoon grated Parmesan cheese; pour over vegetables. Cover and cook 3 minutes. Serve with mini whole-wheat pita.

Blueberry Muffins

Muffins are the next best thing to having cake for breakfast. But as with cake, their buttery sweetness loads you up with calories and fat. Ours—with whole-grain oats and canola oil—are still scrumptious, and they're a healthier way to start the day.

Active time 20 minutes
Total time 45 minutes
plus cooling
Makes 12 muffins

- 1 **cup old-fashioned oats, uncooked**
- 1½ **cups all-purpose flour**
- ½ **cup packed brown sugar**
- 2 **teaspoons baking powder**
- ½ **teaspoon baking soda**
- ½ **teaspoon salt**
- 1 **large egg**
- 1 **cup plus 2 tablespoons buttermilk**
- 3 **tablespoons canola oil**
- 1 **teaspoon vanilla extract**
- 2 **cups blueberries**
- 1 **teaspoon granulated sugar**

1. Preheat oven to 400°F. Spray 12-cup muffin pan with nonstick cooking spray.

2. Place oats in blender and blend until finely ground.

3. In large bowl, combine oats, flour, brown sugar, baking powder and soda, and salt. In small bowl, with fork, blend egg, buttermilk, oil, and vanilla; stir into flour mixture until flour is moistened. Fold in berries.

4. Spoon batter into muffin-pan cups; sprinkle with granulated sugar. Bake 23 to 25 minutes or until toothpick inserted in center of muffins comes out clean. Invert onto wire rack; serve warm, or cool to serve later.

EACH MUFFIN: ABOUT 165 CALORIES, 4 G PROTEIN, 27 G CARBOHYDRATE, 5 G TOTAL FAT (1 G SATURATED), 19 MG CHOLESTEROL, 250 MG SODIUM, 2 G FIBER

Classic Blueberry Muffins
ONE MUFFIN: 270 CALORIES
Healthy Makeover Blueberry Muffins
ONE MUFFIN: 165 CALORIES

You Save **105** CALORIES

Make It a Drop 5 Meal

Serve 1 muffin with sausage links totaling 160 calories, such as 4 Jimmy Dean turkey sausage links or, for a vegetarian option, 2 Morningstar Farms veggie sausage patties. Add ½ grapefruit.
COMPLETE MEAL: 350 CALORIES

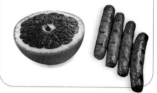

breakfast

Sunday-Morning Omelets

5 EASY FILLINGS

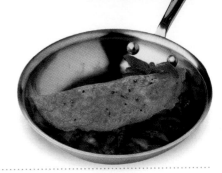

Basic Omelet: In medium bowl, with wire whisk, beat 8 large eggs, ½ cup water, and ½ teaspoon salt. In nonstick 10-inch skillet, melt 1 teaspoon trans-fat-free margarine over medium-high heat. Pour ½ cup egg mixture into skillet. Cook, gently lifting edge of eggs with heat-safe rubber spatula and tilting pan to allow uncooked eggs to run underneath, until eggs are set, about 1 minute. Spoon chosen filling (see below) over half of omelet. Fold unfilled omelet half over filling and slide onto warm plate. Repeat 4 times. Makes 4 servings.

1 Black Bean and Salsa

In nonstick 10-inch skillet, cook 1 cup canned black beans (rinsed and drained) and 1 cup salsa over medium-high heat, stirring frequently until liquid has evaporated. Remove from heat and mix in 1 ripe medium avocado, peeled and chopped, and divide among 4 omelets.

1 OMELET: 362 CALORIES

Make It a Drop 5 Meal
Top with 1 tablespoon reduced-fat sour cream.

385 COMPLETE MEAL CALORIES

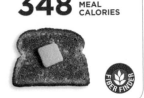

2 Garden Vegetables

In nonstick 10-inch skillet, heat 1 tablespoon olive oil over medium heat. Add 1 small onion, chopped; 1 small zucchini, chopped; 1 small yellow pepper, chopped; ½ teaspoon salt; and ⅛ teaspoon ground black pepper. Cook until vegetables are tender, about 10 minutes. Stir in 2 ripe plum tomatoes, chopped, and ¼ cup chopped fresh basil. Heat through and divide among 4 omelets.

1 OMELET: 234 CALORIES

Make It a Drop 5 Meal
Pair with 1 slice whole-wheat toast spread with 1 teaspoon trans-fat-free margarine.

348 COMPLETE MEAL CALORIES

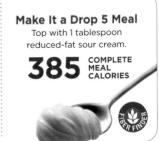

3 Red Pepper and Goat Cheese

In nonstick 10-inch skillet, melt 2 teaspoons trans-fat-free margarine over medium-high heat. Add 1 red pepper, thinly sliced, and ¼ teaspoon salt; cook until tender and lightly browned. Add 1 garlic clove, finely chopped; cook 1 minute. Divide sautéed pepper, 2 ounces plain goat cheese, and ½ cup torn arugula among 4 omelets.

1 OMELET: 249 CALORIES

Make It a Drop 5 Meal
Pair with 1½ cups raspberries.

345 COMPLETE MEAL CALORIES

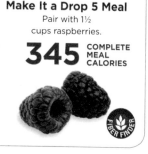

4 Western Style

In nonstick 10-inch skillet, heat 1 tablespoon olive oil over medium heat. Add 1 small onion, chopped; 1 green pepper, chopped; 8 ounces mushrooms, sliced; and ¼ teaspoon salt. Cook until vegetables are tender and liquid has evaporated, about 10 minutes. Add 4 ounces lean ham, finely chopped (about 1 cup), and heat through. Divide among 4 omelets.

1 OMELET: 320 CALORIES

Make It a Drop 5 Meal
Pair with ½ cup cubed melon.

348 COMPLETE MEAL CALORIES

5 Spinach, Cheese, and Bacon

Wash, dry, and remove tough stems from 1 bunch or 10-ounce bag prewashed spinach. In 3-quart saucepan, cook over high heat just until wilted; drain. When cool enough to handle, squeeze out excess liquid from spinach and coarsely chop. Divide spinach; 2 ounces reduced-fat cheddar cheese, shredded; and 3 slices bacon, cooked and crumbled, among 4 omelets.

1 OMELET: 315 CALORIES

Make It a Drop 5 Meal
Pair with ½ grapefruit.

356 COMPLETE MEAL CALORIES

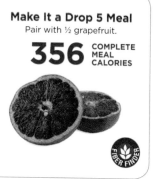

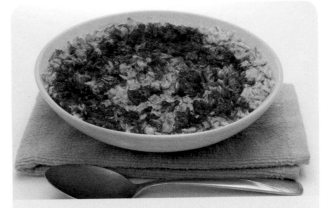

Make Your Own Café au Lait

Mix 1 cup brewed coffee with 1 cup heated fat-free milk; add a sprinkle of cinnamon or cocoa powder for sweet flavor, if desired.

Or you can whip up a low-fat latte instead—even if you don't have an espresso machine at home. Combine 1 to 2 ounces powdered espresso with 1 cup fat-free milk; heat in the microwave for 1 minute.

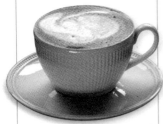

Starbucks Grande Mocha
360 CALORIES
Homemade Café au Lait
90 CALORIES

You Save
270
CALORIES

An Instant Success

Oatmeal with snazzy mix-ins have become a popular pick at places like Starbucks and McDonald's. Try this winner at home, with these yummy additions. Prepare 1 cup cooked plain oatmeal (regular, quick, or instant) with water as package label directs and add:

- ¼ cup shredded apple and a few pinches pumpkin-pie spice **182 TOTAL CALORIES**

- ½ banana and 1 tablespoon mini chocolate chips **282 TOTAL CALORIES**

- 1 tablespoon dried cranberries, 1 tablespoon chopped walnuts, and 1 teaspoon maple syrup **252 TOTAL CALORIES**

- 1 tablespoon each sunflower seeds, dried pineapple, and toasted coconut **261 TOTAL CALORIES**

- 1 tablespoon honey and ½ teaspoon prepared chai spice blend—or your own combo of cardamom, cinnamon, ginger, cloves, and pepper **230 TOTAL CALORIES**

HEALTHY RECIPE MAKEOVER
French Toast

Our slimmed-down take on this Sunday-morning family favorite is practically saintly. Using low-fat milk and egg whites gives it half the fat of traditional French toast. Plus, it's a cinch to whip up.

Active time 10 minutes
Total time 23 minutes
Makes 4 servings

- 2 **large egg whites**
- 1 **large egg**
- ¾ **cup low-fat (1%) milk**
- ¼ **teaspoon vanilla extract**
- ½ **teaspoon salt**
- 2 **teaspoons butter or trans-fat-free margarine**
- 8 **slices firm whole-wheat bread**

1. Preheat oven to 200°F. In pie plate, with whisk, beat egg whites, egg, milk, vanilla, and salt until blended. In 12-inch nonstick skillet, melt 1 teaspoon butter or trans-fat-free margarine on medium heat.

2. Dip bread slices, one at a time, in egg mixture, pressing bread lightly to coat both sides well. Place 3 or 4 slices in skillet, and cook 3 to 4 minutes or until lightly browned; flip and cook 3 to 4 minutes on second side.

3. Transfer French toast to cookie sheet; keep warm in oven. Repeat with remaining butter or margarine, bread slices, and egg mixture.

EACH 2-SLICE SERVING: ABOUT 300 CALORIES, 12 G PROTEIN, 46 G CARBOHYDRATE, 9 G TOTAL FAT (2 G SATURATED), 56 MG CHOLESTEROL, 755 MG SODIUM, 6 G FIBER

Classic French toast
SINGLE SERVING: 570 CALORIES
Healthy Makeover French Toast
SINGLE SERVING: 300 CALORIES

You Save
270
CALORIES

Make It a Drop 5 Meal
Serve with ½ cup berries and 1 tablespoon maple syrup
COMPLETE MEAL: 384 CALORIES

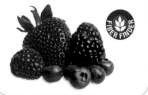

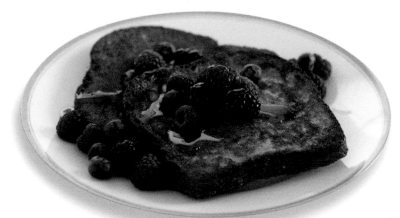

GIVE YOUR
lunch a lift

What do you do when you find yourself at home at lunchtime? Do you go for your kids' PB & J fixings? Or maybe you skip lunch completely and end up snacking all afternoon. Here are some midday meal ideas for when you're homebound and trying to Drop 5. (See also page 116 for eating lunch at the office and page 118 for dining out.)

Eat Vegetarian Once a Week

Swap veggies for meat for lunch just once a week and you could Drop 5 (or more) in a year. When Johns Hopkins researchers fed 54 men and women similar lunches (one mushroom-based, the other beef-based), they consumed roughly 30 fewer grams of fat per day when they went veggie—and found the mushroom meal as satisfying as the meat. Not a fan of mushrooms? Subbing a low-cal, high-fiber vegetarian meal, like a veggie burger or the Dijon Bean and Veggie Salad, opposite, may also do the trick.

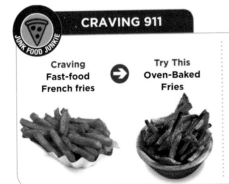

CRAVING 911

Craving Fast-food French fries ➔ **Try This Oven-Baked Fries**

Preheat oven to 425°F. Toss 1 unpeeled baking potato (about 5 ounces), cut into wedges, with 1 teaspoon oil and a sprinkle of salt. Arrange in single layer in shallow pan. Bake 25 minutes, turning once, until potatoes are golden.

Large order fast-food French fries (5 ounces)
500 CALORIES
Oven-Baked Fries (5 ounces)
145 CALORIES

You Save 355 CALORIES

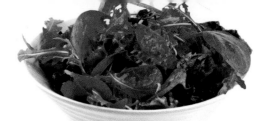

TOP 5 LUNCH SALADS

 These easy-to-toss-together salads will keep your calories low and fiber and satisfaction levels high.

1. **DIJON BEAN AND VEGGIE SALAD** In medium bowl, combine ½ cup each canned (rinsed and drained) kidney beans and garbanzo beans. Add ½ cup sliced cucumbers, ½ cup chopped tomatoes, and ½ cup sliced carrots. Toss with 2 teaspoons olive oil, 2 tablespoons cider vinegar, 1 teaspoon Dijon mustard, 1 minced garlic clove, ¼ teaspoon ground cumin, and ¼ teaspoon ground black pepper. Serve with 6 Triscuit crackers. **513 TOTAL CALORIES**

2. **CHICKEN AND RICE SALAD** Combine ½ cup cooked brown rice with ¾ cup diced cooked chicken breast, ⅓ cup shredded carrots, and ½ cup chopped broccoli. Toss with 1 teaspoon sesame oil, 2 tablespoons lemon juice, 1 minced garlic clove, and 2 teaspoons light soy sauce. Serve with 1 cup pineapple chunks. **460 TOTAL CALORIES**

3. **HONEY MUSTARD CHICKEN SALAD** Toss 3 cups mixed greens with ½ cup each sliced sweet onion, sliced cucumbers, shredded carrots, and grape tomatoes. Top with 2 tablespoons shredded reduced-fat cheddar or Monterey Jack cheese, 2 tablespoons store-bought honey-mustard dressing, and 1 cup chopped or sliced boneless skinless chicken breast (can be pulled from rotisserie chicken). Serve with 1 small piece of fruit, such as a tangerine or plum. **494 TOTAL CALORIES**

4. **LIME TUNA AND BLACK BEAN SALAD** Toss 3 cups mixed greens with ½ cup each sliced cucumbers, sliced sweet onion, corn, and canned black beans (rinsed and drained), as well as ¼ avocado, sliced. Toss with 2 tablespoons store-bought lime dressing (such as Newman's Own Light Lime Vinaigrette) and top with 3 ounces tuna from can or pouch. **498 TOTAL CALORIES**

5. **SWEET AND SAVORY SALMON SALAD** Toss 3 cups mixed greens with ½ cup each sliced cucumber and sliced strawberries, ¼ cup each mandarin oranges and feta cheese, 2 tablespoons dried cranberries, and 1 tablespoon sliced almonds. Toss with 2 tablespoons store-bought red wine vinaigrette and top with 3 ounces salmon from can or pouch. **512 TOTAL CALORIES**

The 450-Calorie Sandwich

A sandwich doesn't have to be loaded with fat and calories, especially when you're making it at home. Here's how to construct the perfect in-house sandwich in a snap.

- **BREAD: 200 CALORIES** Choose whole-grain bread for your sandwich—but watch the size. A big sub roll, for example, might have up to 500 calories! Instead, choose two slices of whole-grain or whole-wheat sandwich bread or one small roll equal to about 200 calories.

- **CHEESE: 50 CALORIES** You can add cheese to your sandwich without breaking the calorie bank: One slice of reduced-fat Sargento pepper Jack, for example, is only 50 calories. Look for any variety of reduced-fat cheese with about 50 calories and no more than 3 or 4 fat grams per slice.

- **MEAT: 100 CALORIES** Many luncheon meats are high in calories and sodium. Cured meat or sausage sandwiches should be occasional indulgences, not everyday fare. Look for lower-calorie alternatives such as chicken breast, roast beef, turkey breast, ham, and water-packed tuna. Aim for about 100 calories of lean protein, which is about 5 slices of meat (each deli slice is around 20 calories) or a 3-ounce can of tuna in water.

- **SPREADS: 50 CALORIES** Instead of high-fat mayonnaise, use one of the reduced-fat varieties and add some chopped fresh herbs for flavor. Or hold the mayo and spread your bread with naturally low-fat mustard; specialty food stores carry a wide selection. For a creamier version, make a spread of nonfat yogurt mixed with a bit of mustard. Chutney or relish, delicious by itself or when blended with light mayonnaise or mustard, adds a delectable sweet-and-spicy dimension to a sandwich.

- **VEGGIES: NO LIMIT** Go wild—add spinach, lettuce, red pepper, onions, cucumber, jalapeños, mushrooms, tomato, or any other fresh vegetable to any sandwich for extra flavor, fiber, and virtually no calories. Avoid veggies packed or roasted in oil; they also pack unwanted calories. And go easy on the avocado (58 calories per ¼ cup sliced)—a little goes a long way.

TOTAL CALORIE GOAL: AROUND 450
Now, to finish your meal, add a piece of fruit (a banana, pear, or nectarine, for example). Voilà—the perfect lunch to help you Drop 5!

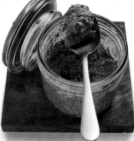

THE SKINNY ON SANDWICH SPREADS

SPREAD	GRAMS FAT	CALORIES PER TABLESPOON
Mayonnaise	10	90
Pesto	7	75
Ranch dressing	7.5	73
Light mayonnaise	4.5	45
Italian dressing	4	43
Honey mustard	0	30
Barbecue sauce	0	24
Hummus	1.5	23
Relish or chutney	0	20
Ketchup	0	15
Mustard	0.5	9
Salsa	0	5

HEALTHY RECIPE MAKEOVER
Tuna Salad

That deli and diner staple, tuna salad, may be tasty and convenient, but it's not always the healthiest meal choice.

Proof: One popular sandwich-shop version has more than a third of your daily fat quota—24 grams, 4 of which are saturated fats—in a mere ⅓ cup. A serving of our remake is almost double the size, with a fat tally that's 18 grams slimmer, thanks to a mix of low-fat mayo and nonfat yogurt. Plus, veggies add flavor, crunch, fiber, and vitamins.

Classic tuna salad
SINGLE SERVING: 240 CALORIES
Healthy Makeover Tuna Salad
SINGLE SERVING: 135 CALORIES

You Save
105
CALORIES

Make It a Drop 5 Meal
Serve on 2 slices bread topped with 2 leaves green lettuce and 2 slices tomato. Pair with 1½ cups canned lentil soup.
COMPLETE MEAL: 511 CALORIES

FIBER FINDER

Total time 15 minutes
Makes about 2½ cups or 4 main-dish servings

- 2 **(5-ounce) cans chunk-light tuna in water, drained**
- 2 **medium stalks celery, chopped**
- 1 **medium carrot, shredded (½ cup)**
- ½ **medium red pepper (4 to 6 ounces), chopped**
- ¼ **cup light mayonnaise**
- 3 **tablespoons nonfat plain yogurt**
- 1 **tablespoon fresh lemon juice**
- ¼ **teaspoon ground black pepper**

In medium bowl, combine tuna, celery, carrot, red pepper, mayonnaise, yogurt, lemon juice, and black pepper.

EACH SERVING: ABOUT 135 CALORIES, 16 G PROTEIN, 6 G CARBOHYDRATE, 6 G TOTAL FAT (1 G SATURATED), 22 MG CHOLESTEROL, 340 MG SODIUM, 1 G FIBER

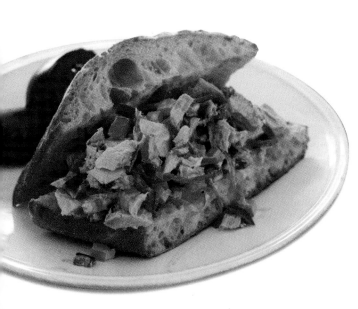

MYTH BUSTER

Fiction Carbs spell trouble for dieters.
Fact Carbohydrates are actually an important source of energy. Even so, that doesn't mean there's nothing to learn from low-carb diets. Carbs are not all created equal, and to help you Drop 5, you want to limit processed carbs such as white bread and croissants. Instead, enjoy beans and whole grains such as brown rice and whole-wheat bread. And don't forget fruits and vegetables, which provide a host of nutrients and fiber, are low in calories, and can help reduce the risk of obesity and heart disease.

The body also uses carbs as fuel during exercise to burn body fat—another great reason to keep bread (and sandwiches!) on the menu.

SIMPLE SWAPS

Swap This
2 TABLESPOONS
FULL-FAT SALAD DRESSING
(ABOUT 150 CALORIES)

For This
10 PUMPS
SPRAY SALAD DRESSING
(ABOUT 10 CALORIES)

You Save
140
CALORIES

Drop 5

DO IT NOW
Have Your Sandwich Open-Faced
By skipping the extra bread, you'll slim down your sandwich.

You Save
100
CALORIES

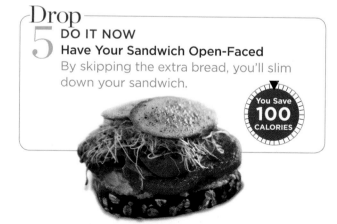

Canned Beans
5 EASY WAYS

Low in fat and high in protein, beans are a quick, delicious route to a healthy lunch at home. Pop open one (or more) 15-ounce cans to make any of these slimming recipes.

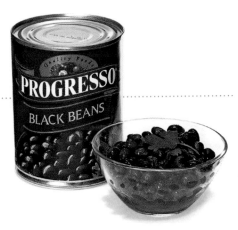

1 Black Bean Dip

In food processor, puree 1 can drained and rinsed black beans with 1 tablespoon fresh lime juice, 1 teaspoon freshly grated lime peel, and 2 teaspoons chipotle pepper sauce. Transfer to small bowl and stir in ¼ cup chopped cilantro leaves and 2 plum tomatoes, seeded and chopped.

MAKES ABOUT 2 CUPS

SERVING SIZE: ½ CUP, 172 CALORIES

Make It a Drop 5 Meal
Serve with a whole-wheat pita (cut into pieces for dipping), 2 cups of your favorite raw vegetables, and for dessert, 1 cup pineapple chunks.

471 COMPLETE MEAL CALORIES

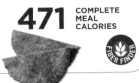

2 Garbanzo Bean Salad

In medium bowl, combine 1 can drained and rinsed garbanzo beans, 1 chopped red pepper, 1 can (15 ¼ ounces) drained corn kernels, ⅓ cup chopped cilantro leaves, and 2 tablespoons ranch dressing.

MAKES ABOUT 3½ CUPS

SERVING SIZE: 1 CUP, 330 CALORIES

Make It a Drop 5 Meal
Serve over a bed of greens and top with ½ cup ripe avocado, cubed. For dessert, have an orange.

522 COMPLETE MEAL CALORIES

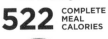
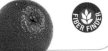

3 Black-Eyed Pea Sauté

In nonstick skillet, brown 1 small onion, chopped, in 1 teaspoon olive oil. Stir in 1 clove garlic, crushed with press, and cook 1 minute. Stir in 1 can drained and rinsed black-eyed peas and heat through. Remove from heat and stir in 1 to 2 tablespoons chopped pickled jalapeño chiles.

MAKES ABOUT 2 CUPS

SERVING SIZE: ½ CUP, 183 CALORIES

Make It a Drop 5 Meal
Top with 1 ounce shredded reduced-fat cheddar cheese and serve with an 8-inch whole-wheat tortilla and an apple.

475 COMPLETE MEAL CALORIES

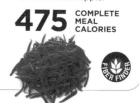

4 Black Bean Soup

In large nonstick saucepan, combine 1 cup salsa and 1 pinch allspice and cook over medium heat for 3 minutes. Stir in 2 cans drained and rinsed black beans and 3 cups low-sodium chicken broth; raise heat to medium-high and bring to boil. Reduce heat and simmer 10 minutes. Use immersion blender or potato masher to coarsely mash beans in the pot.

MAKES ABOUT 6 CUPS

SERVING SIZE: 1 CUP, 240 CALORIES

Make It a Drop 5 Meal
Top with a dollop of reduced-fat sour cream and serve with 2 cups mixed greens tossed with 10 pumps spray dressing, 1 ounce baked tortilla chips (around 17 chips), and a pear.

513 COMPLETE MEAL CALORIES

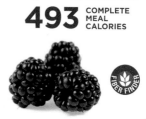

5 Kidney Bean Chili

In large nonstick saucepan, cook 8 ounces lean ground turkey and 1 small onion, chopped, until beef is browned and onion is tender, about 10 minutes. Stir in 2 teaspoons chili powder and cook 1 minute. Stir in 2 cans drained and rinsed kidney beans, 1 can (14 ounces) diced tomatoes with green chiles, and 1 cup water. Heat to boiling over medium-high heat; reduce heat to low and simmer 15 minutes, stirring occasionally.

MAKES ABOUT 5 CUPS

SERVING SIZE: 1 CUP, 363 CALORIES

Make It a Drop 5 Meal
Top with 1 ounce shredded reduced-fat cheddar cheese. Serve with 2 cups mixed greens tossed with 10 pumps spray dressing and ½ cup blackberries.

493 COMPLETE MEAL CALORIES

SELECT SMART
snacks

Think you need to give up snacking to lose weight? On the contrary, the Drop 5 plan has two 100-calorie snacks built right in. Here are our favorites—salty and sweet—to help you Drop 5.

50-CALORIE SALTY SNACKS

These tasty snack ideas will help keep hunger at bay, and at around 50 calories, you can have two to four per day.

1. 1 Ak-Mak Stone Ground Whole Wheat Sesame Cracker with 1 tablespoon mashed avocado
2. 1½ tablespoons hummus with ½ small red pepper, sliced, for dipping
3. 1 tablespoon soft herbed goat cheese with 1 stalk celery
4. 10 baby carrots with 2 tablespoons salsa for dipping
5. 20 thin pretzels with 1 tablespoon Dijon mustard for dipping

50-CALORIE SWEET SNACKS

Satisfy your sugar cravings with these quick, low-cal fixes.

1. 1 Jell-O sugar-free pudding cup (any flavor)
2. 6 chocolate or vanilla Miss Meringue Minis
3. 1 Breyers All Natural Pure Fruit Bar
4. 14 frozen grapes
5. ⅓ cup fresh raspberries drizzled with 1 teaspoon melted chocolate chips

The 100-Calorie Comparison Low-density

foods have relatively few calories compared with what they weigh. These foods are high in water or fiber and add bulk to your meals, so you feel satisfied with fewer calories. For example, all the foods below can be diet-friendly snacks, but the strawberries will leave you feeling the fullest.

 = = 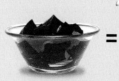 =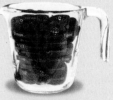

| 23 M&M's | ¼ cup raisins | 5 ounces of regular Jell-O | 2¼ cups strawberries |

Drop

5 DO IT NOW Stock Your House with Calorie-Controlled Snacks

Calorie-controlled packs of your favorite not-so-healthy snacks make it easier for you to indulge without overdoing it. Store shelves are chock-full of **100-calorie packs of cookies, chips, crackers,** snack cakes, brownies, and more. While they cost more than larger bags of the same snack, they cost less than a larger size pair of pants.

Plus, **think of them as training wheels for dieting**: 100-calorie snack packs can help you learn how to keep indulgences in check. In a University of Colorado Denver study, 59 adults ate snack foods for two weeks. Half the group munched from 100-calorie bags for one week, followed by the same treats from large bags for the next; for the other half, the order was reversed. **Outcome:** Volunteers who were first "trained" with small packs took 852 fewer calories from the big bags. You can learn to **recognize the right amount,** say the study authors, who suggest eating the 100-calorie size (or measuring out that amount) of a favorite. Then, whenever you encounter that snack food, **you'll know what a "safe" portion is.**

snacks

100-CALORIE MUNCHIES

Each of these tasty nibbles has around 100 calories, so you can have one or two a day.

(Note: Yellow highlights indicate foods shown in photographs.)

SWEET TREATS

- 1 Whole Foods Market Two-Bite Brownie
- 1 Kozy Shack Simply Well pudding cup (any flavor)
- 1 Healthy Choice Mocha Swirl Bar
- 1 pouch Keebler Sandies Right Bites Shortbread Cookies
- ½ cup Sharon's Lemon Sorbet with ¼ cup blueberries
- 1 Nestlé Skinny Cow 98% Fat-Free Fudge Bar
- 1 Nestlé Butterfinger Stixx Candy
- 5 Nabisco Nilla Wafers
- 3 Country Choice Organic Ginger Snaps
- 1 Deep Chocolate VitaMuffin VitaTop
- 1 Blue Bunny FrozFruit Chunky Pineapple Bar

FRUITS AND VEGGIES

- 2 cups raspberries
- 1 cup mango slices
- 4 strawberries with 4 tablespoons Cool Whip for dipping
- 1 cup grapes
- 1 cup blueberries
- ½ medium cantaloupe
- ½ small apple with 2 teaspoons peanut butter
- 45 steamed edamame pods (green soybeans)
- 2 tablespoons each mashed avocado and chopped tomatoes stuffed in ½ mini pita

SIMPLE SWAPS

Swap This
150 CALORIES PER CUP WHOLE MILK

For This
90 CALORIES PER CUP SKIM MILK

LIQUID CALORIE LOVER

Milk

You Save
60
CALORIES

DAIRY DELIGHTS

- 1 Organic Valley Part-Skim Mozzarella Stringles String Cheese
- ¼ cup low-fat cottage cheese with ½ cup canned peaches without added sugar or 2 canned pear halves or 2 canned pineapple slices
- 1 Laughing Cow Light Garlic & Herb Cheese Wedge and 3 Triscuits
- 6 ounces nonfat plain yogurt topped with ⅓ cup raspberries

SAVORY BITES

- 20 roasted peanuts
- 60 Pepperidge Farm Baby Goldfish Crackers
- 1 Jolly Time Healthy Pop Mini Bag of Popcorn
- 12 Back to Nature Sesame Ginger Rice Thins
- 40 Rold Gold Classic Style Pretzel Sticks
- 12 Quaker Quakes Cheddar Cheese Rice Snacks
- 20 Glenny's Low-Fat Soy Crisps
- 10 Guiltless Gourmet Baked Yellow Corn Chips with ¼ cup salsa

HEARTY HELPINGS

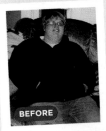

- 1 Campbell's Soup at Hand Blended Vegetable Medley
- 1 Nature Valley Crunchy Granola Bar
- 1 hard-boiled egg with 1 slice melba toast
- 4 slices thin-sliced deli ham with 2 teaspoons honey mustard, rolled in lettuce leaf
- 1 slice Pepperidge Farm Swirl Raisin Cinnamon Bread with 1 teaspoon trans-fat-free margarine
- ½ mini bagel with 1 ounce smoked salmon
- 1 Kellogg's Eggo Nutri-Grain Low Fat Whole Grain Waffle with 1 tablespoon Smucker's Squeeze Fruit Spread

Learn from the "Losers"

"I used to start snacking as soon as I got home from work. Now, I change into my workout clothes and head right back out for a quick run."

—JAN HAAPALA, 130 POUNDS LOST

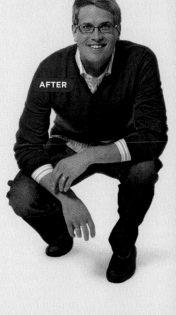

BEFORE

AFTER

MAKE DINNER
a winner

At about 500 calories each, the delicious dinners in this section will help you lose weight and keep you satisfied, too.

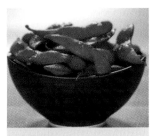

MAKE IT A HABIT

Eat Veggies or Salad as a First Course

Try this: Before dinner, open a bag of frozen edamame (green soybeans), zap them in the microwave, and serve them, still in the pod, as a starter. Or begin your meal with a simple mixed green salad with a few pumps of low-cal spray dressing. You're likely to eat much less at the meal.

Going with the Grain

Dutch researchers surveyed more than 4,000 people and found that those who ate just one serving a day of whole grains weighed about seven pounds less than those who didn't. Why? Whole grains, which are high in fiber, digest so slowly you feel full longer; that means you're likely to eat less and, therefore, lose more.

Nearly every supermarket now carries even exotic varieties of grains like quinoa and wheat berries (whole-grain wheat). Stock up, then store your supplies in tightly covered containers and refrigerate them during the warmer months. And don't forget about whole-grain spaghetti, whole-wheat couscous, brown rice, and other faves! For recipe ideas, see "Whole-Grain Pasta 5 Easy Ways," page 58.

Meat Loaf

In the kingdom of comfort food, meat loaf is royalty. To get the comfort without the calories, try this version, made with 93 percent lean ground turkey.

Active time 15 minutes
Total time 1 hour 10 minutes plus standing
Makes 8 main-dish servings

- 1 **tablespoon olive oil**
- 2 **medium stalks celery, finely chopped**
- 1 **small onion, finely chopped**
- 1 **clove garlic, crushed with press**
- 2 **pounds lean ground turkey**
- ¾ **cup (from 1½ slices bread) fresh whole-wheat bread crumbs**
- ⅓ **cup fat-free milk**
- 1 **tablespoon Worcestershire sauce**
- 2 **large egg whites**
- ½ **cup ketchup**
- ½ **teaspoon salt**
- ¼ **teaspoon coarsely ground black pepper**
- 1 **tablespoon Dijon mustard**

1. Preheat oven to 350°F. In 12-inch nonstick skillet, heat oil on medium and cook celery and onion 10 minutes or until tender, stirring occasionally. Add garlic and cook 1 minute. Transfer vegetables to large bowl; cool slightly.

2. To bowl with vegetables, add turkey, bread crumbs, milk, Worcestershire sauce, egg whites, ¼ cup ketchup, salt, and pepper; mix with hands until well combined but not overmixed. In cup, combine Dijon and remaining ¼ cup ketchup.

3. In 13" by 9" metal baking pan, shape meat mixture into 9" by 5" loaf. (This will allow meat loaf to brown all over, not just on top.) Spread ketchup mixture over top of loaf.

4. Bake meat loaf 55 to 60 minutes or until meat thermometer inserted in center reaches 160°F. (Temperature will rise to 165°F upon standing.)

5. Let meat loaf stand 10 minutes before removing from pan to set juices for easier slicing. Transfer meat loaf to platter and serve.

EACH SERVING: ABOUT 230 CALORIES, 25 G PROTEIN, 11 G CARBOHYDRATE, 11 G TOTAL FAT (3 G SATURATED), 80 MG CHOLESTEROL, 500 MG SODIUM, 1 G FIBER

Classic meat loaf
SINGLE SERVING: 470 CALORIES
Healthy Makeover Meat Loaf
SINGLE SERVING: 230 CALORIES

You Save
240
CALORIES

Make It a Drop 5 Dinner
Serve with a small baked potato topped with 1 tablespoon trans-fat-free margarine and 10 spears of steamed asparagus
COMPLETE MEAL: 483 CALORIES

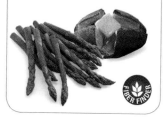

Whole-Grain Pasta
5 EASY WAYS

For a meal to serve four, prepare 4 cups cooked whole-grain pasta as package label directs (2 ounces uncooked pasta yields 1 to 2 cups cooked pasta, depending on the shape). Serve with any of these figure-friendly sauces. For a balanced and filling meal, make pasta the side dish and fill the rest of your plate with lean protein and veggies.

1 Confetti Pasta

In 10-inch skillet, heat 2 teaspoons olive oil over medium heat. Add 2 carrots, shredded; 1 medium zucchini (8 ounces), shredded; 1 garlic clove, crushed with garlic press; ¾ teaspoon salt; and ¼ teaspoon coarsely ground black pepper; cook 5 minutes. Stir in cooked pasta; heat through.

SERVING SIZE: 1 CUP PASTA, 219 CALORIES

Make It a Drop 5 Meal
Top with 1 tablespoon grated Parmesan cheese and pair with 6 ounces grilled shrimp and 2 cups mixed greens tossed with 10 pumps spray dressing

453 COMPLETE MEAL CALORIES

FIBER FINDER

2 Orange-Fennel Pasta

In 10-inch skillet, heat 2 teaspoons olive oil over medium heat. Add 1 garlic clove, crushed with garlic press; ¾ teaspoon salt; and ¼ teaspoon coarsely ground black pepper and cook 30 seconds. Stir in 1 teaspoon freshly grated orange peel and ½ teaspoon fennel seeds, crushed. Stir in cooked pasta and 2 tablespoons chopped fresh parsley; heat through.

SERVING SIZE: 1 CUP PASTA, 197 CALORIES

Make It a Drop 5 Meal
Serve with 3 ounces baked or grilled pork tenderloin, 1 cup spinach sautéed with chopped garlic and 1 teaspoon olive oil, and 2 cups mixed greens tossed with 10 pumps spray dressing

463 COMPLETE MEAL CALORIES

FIBER FINDER

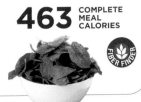

3 Pasta with Peas and Onion

In 10-inch skillet, heat 2 teaspoons olive oil over medium heat. Add 1 small onion, chopped, and 2 tablespoons water and cook until onion is tender and golden, about 10 minutes. Stir in cooked pasta and 1 cup frozen peas, thawed; heat through.

SERVING SIZE: 1 CUP PASTA, 232 CALORIES

Make It a Drop 5 Meal

Top with 1 tablespoon grated Parmesan cheese and serve with 3 ounces broiled salmon and 2 cups mixed greens tossed with 10 pumps spray dressing

459 COMPLETE MEAL CALORIES

---

4 Pasta with Tomatoes and Lemon

In serving bowl, combine 2 pounds ripe tomatoes; ¼ cup loosely packed fresh mint leaves, chopped; ¼ cup loosely packed fresh basil leaves, chopped; 1 garlic clove, crushed with garlic press; 1 teaspoon freshly grated lemon peel; 2 tablespoons olive oil; 1 teaspoon salt; and ¼ teaspoon ground black pepper. Let stand at least 15 minutes or up to 1 hour at room temperature to blend flavors. Add pasta to tomato mixture and toss well.

SERVING SIZE: 1 CUP PASTA, 310 CALORIES

Make It a Drop 5 Meal

Top with 3 ounces baked or grilled sliced chicken breast and serve with 2 cups mixed greens tossed with 10 pumps spray dressing

COMPLETE MEAL CALORIES

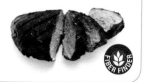

---

5 Marinara Pasta

In nonreactive 3-quart saucepan, heat 2 tablespoons olive oil over medium heat; add 1 small onion, chopped, and 1 garlic clove, finely chopped, and cook, stirring, until onion is tender, about 5 minutes. Stir in 1 can (28 ounces) plum tomatoes with their juice, 2 tablespoons tomato paste, 2 tablespoons finely chopped fresh basil, and ½ teaspoon salt. Heat to boiling, breaking up tomatoes with side of spoon. Reduce heat; partially cover and simmer, stirring occasionally, until sauce has thickened slightly, about 20 minutes.

SERVING SIZE: 1 CUP PASTA WITH 1 CUP OF THE SAUCE, 208 CALORIES

Make It a Drop 5 Meal

Serve with 3 ounces baked or grilled chicken and 2 cups steamed chopped broccoli topped with 2 tablespoons grated Parmesan cheese

COMPLETE MEAL CALORIES

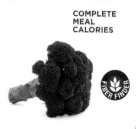

SIMPLE SWAPS

Swap This
360 CALORIES PER BAGEL

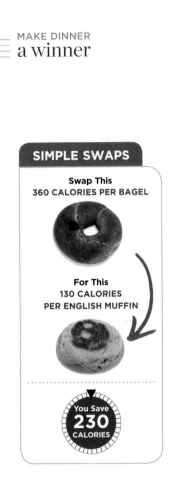

For This
130 CALORIES
PER ENGLISH MUFFIN

You Save
230
CALORIES

Slice It Right

We love pizza, you love pizza, your family loves pizza—but it can be loaded with calories. How to order take-out pizza without ruining your efforts to Drop 5? Top of the list: Lose the high-cal extras such as sausage and pepperoni. Instead, ask for extra veggies—they'll help fill you up. For the most slimming slices, go for the thin crust and ask the pizzeria to use half the normal amount of cheese. You might even try a pie with no cheese; just a sprinkle of Parmesan on top.

At Pizza Hut, you could save 150 calories per slice by switching from the Meat Lover's pan pizza to the Veggie Lover's pizza with the Thin 'N Crispy crust.

330 VERSUS 180 CALORIES

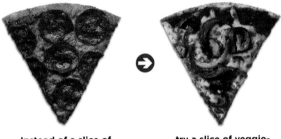

Instead of a slice of meat-topped pan pizza...

...try a slice of veggie-loaded thin-crust pizza

Drop

5 DO IT NOW Spice up Your Meals Research has shown that **fiery flavors** can have long-lasting **weight-reduction benefits.** For example, capsaicin, a compound found in jalapeño, cayenne, and other spicy peppers, can be a powerful **appetite suppressant,** metabolism booster, and fat burner. A Canadian study found that people who ate appetizers made with hot pepper consumed 189 **fewer calories** at their next meal. Not a fan of spicy foods? Zero-calorie herbs are also a great way to **punch up** the flavor in a dish.

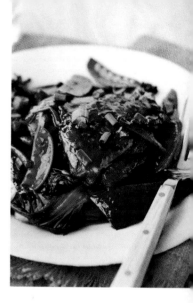

Red-Cooked Chicken with Assorted Vegetables

A sweet and spicy glaze wraps this richly hued Asian-style chicken, which practically falls off the bone, thanks to gentle simmering in a slow cooker. And, at just 355 calories per serving, it's a protein- and fiber-packed Drop 5 star.

Active time 20 minutes
Total time 8 hours on Low or 4 hours on High
Makes 4 main-dish servings

- ½ **cup dry sherry**
- ⅓ **cup low-sodium soy sauce**
- ¼ **cup packed brown sugar**
- 2 **tablespoons grated peeled fresh ginger**
- 1 **teaspoon Chinese five-spice powder**
- 3 **garlic cloves, crushed with press**
- 1 **bunch green onions, cut into 2-inch pieces (white and green parts separated)**
- 3 **pounds bone-in skinless chicken thighs**
- 1 **bag (16 ounces) assorted fresh veggies for stir-fry (such as snow peas, carrots, broccoli, and red pepper)**

1. In 5- to 6-quart slow cooker, combine sherry, soy sauce, brown sugar, ginger, five-spice powder, garlic, and white parts of green onions. Add chicken thighs and toss to coat with sherry mixture. Cover slow cooker and cook as manufacturer directs, on Low 8 hours or on High 4 hours.

2. Coarsely chop remaining green onion parts; wrap and refrigerate until serving time.

3. Just before serving, place vegetables in microwave-safe medium bowl and cook in microwave as label directs.

4. With tongs, transfer chicken to deep platter. Stir vegetables into slow cooker to coat with sauce. Spoon vegetable mixture around chicken. Sprinkle with reserved green onions.

EACH SERVING: ABOUT 355 CALORIES, 43 G PROTEIN, 27 G CARBOHYDRATE, 8 G TOTAL FAT (2 G SATURATED), 161 MG CHOLESTEROL, 881 MG SODIUM, 4 G FIBER

Slow Cook to Weight Loss

Slow cookers do all the work and give you all the credit for their saucy, warming suppers. Slow-cooked dishes are ideal for making ahead and reheating, and provide leftovers for several days. A slow cooker also offers advantages for lower-calorie cooking by stretching small amounts of meat with flavorful sauces and generous amounts of vegetables.

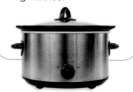

a winner

Chicken Breasts
5 EASY WAYS

Skinless, boneless chicken breasts are the darling of cooks looking to cut fat and calories. This recipe scores, thanks to a choice of easy sauces. In nonstick 12-inch skillet, heat 1 teaspoon vegetable oil over medium heat until very hot. Add 4 small skinless, boneless chicken breast halves (4 to 5 ounces each) and cook until chicken is golden brown and loses its pink color throughout, 4 to 5 minutes per side. Remove chicken from pan and reduce heat to medium, then make one of these sauces.

1 Apple-Curry Sauce

Add 2 teaspoons vegetable oil to skillet. Add 1 Golden Delicious apple, peeled, cored, and sliced, and 1 small onion, sliced. Cook, stirring, until tender. Stir in 1½ teaspoons curry powder and ¼ teaspoon salt; cook 1 minute. Stir in ½ cup mango chutney and ½ cup water. Heat to boiling; boil 1 minute. Spoon equally over chicken breasts.

SERVING SIZE: 1 BREAST WITH ¼ OF THE SAUCE, 342 CALORIES
(Note: Recipe shown in photo above.)

Make It a Drop 5 Meal
Pair with ½ cup cooked wild rice and 1 cup steamed broccoli with 1 teaspoon trans-fat-free margarine

487 COMPLETE MEAL CALORIES

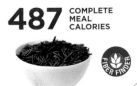

2 Dijon Sauce

Add ½ cup light cream or nonfat half-and-half, 2 tablespoons Dijon mustard with seeds, and ¾ cup seedless red or green grapes, each cut in half, to skillet. Cook over low heat, stirring to blend flavors, until sauce has thickened, about 1 minute. Spoon equally over chicken breasts.

SERVING SIZE: 1 BREAST WITH ¼ OF THE SAUCE, 234 CALORIES

Make It a Drop 5 Meal
Pair with 1 baked sweet potato topped with 1 tablespoon trans-fat-free margarine and 1 cup fresh green beans sautéed with 1 teaspoon olive oil

495 COMPLETE MEAL CALORIES

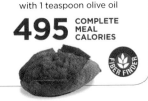

3 Chinese Ginger Sauce

Add 1 teaspoon vegetable oil to skillet. Add 1 red pepper, thinly sliced, and cook until tender-crisp. Add ½ cup water, 2 tablespoons soy sauce, 2 tablespoons seasoned rice vinegar, and 1 tablespoon grated, peeled fresh ginger. Heat to boiling; boil 1 minute. Sprinkle with 2 chopped green onions. Spoon equally over chicken breasts.

SERVING SIZE: 1 BREAST WITH ¼ OF THE SAUCE, 195 CALORIES

Make It a Drop 5 Meal
Pair with 1 cup cooked soba noodles and 1½ cups steamed snow peas drizzled with 1 teaspoon sesame oil. For dessert, have 1 orange.

485 COMPLETE MEAL CALORIES

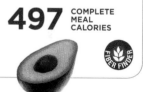

4 Black Bean Salsa

Add 1 can (15 to 19 ounces) black beans, rinsed and drained; 1 jar (10 ounces) thick-and-chunky salsa; 1 can (8¾ ounces) whole-kernel corn, drained; 2 tablespoons chopped fresh cilantro; and ¼ cup water to skillet. Cook, stirring, until heated through, about 1 minute. Spoon equally over chicken breasts.

SERVING SIZE: 1 BREAST WITH ¼ OF THE SAUCE, 282 CALORIES

Make It a Drop 5 Meal
Pair with 2 (6-inch) whole-wheat tortillas; ¼ avocado, mashed; 2 tablespoons shredded reduced-fat cheddar cheese; and 2 cups shredded lettuce.

497 COMPLETE MEAL CALORIES

5 Provençal Sauce

Add 1 teaspoon olive oil or vegetable oil to skillet. Add 1 medium onion, chopped, and cook, stirring, until tender. Stir in 1 can (14½ ounces) Italian-style stewed tomatoes, ½ cup pitted ripe olives (each cut in half), 1 tablespoon drained capers, and ¼ cup water. Cook, stirring, until heated through, about 1 minute. Spoon equally over chicken breasts.

SERVING SIZE: 1 BREAST WITH ¼ OF THE SAUCE, 253 CALORIES

Make It a Drop 5 Meal
Serve over 1 cup cooked whole-wheat couscous alongside 2 cups mixed salad greens tossed with 10 pumps spray dressing.

508 COMPLETE MEAL CALORIES

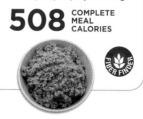

MAKE IT A HABIT
Keep a Food Diary

While you may believe you're eating right, memory is selective. Plus, it's easy to overlook bites, licks, and tastes, but each mouthful has 25 calories, on average. Translation: Six little bites a day add up to around 15 extra pounds a year. The solution is to write it down. In a landmark Kaiser Permanente study of more than 2,000 dieters, keeping a food diary turned out to be the best predictor of whether people would lose weight. So buy a journal and use it every day.

You Say Tomato, We Say Weight Loss

The new diet drink of choice may be veggie juice, report Baylor College of Medicine scientists. When they studied 81 overweight adults who were following the DASH diet (rich in foods like fruits, veggies, whole grains, and lean meats), they found that those who had a daily eight-ounce glass of low-sodium veggie juice lost an average of four pounds in twelve weeks—while a control group lost only one pound. They theorize that the juice, usually tomato mixed with a variety of vegetables, may fill you up so you eat less overall. Try sipping a glass as you cook dinner; you'll get a dose of veggies, and it may stop premeal noshing. Just be sure to work it into your Daily Calorie Target (page 30).

CRAVING 911

Craving		Try This
Pot pie with a side of mashed potatoes	→	**Turkey Mock-Pie**

In saucepan, combine ¾ cup 98-percent-fat-free condensed cream of mushroom soup; ¾ cup bite-size pieces cooked, skinless turkey breast; ¾ cup frozen peas and diced carrots; and 2 tablespoons nonfat milk. Heat to boiling, then spoon into a broiler-safe 3-cup dish. Top with ⅔ cup ready-to-heat mashed potatoes; broil until lightly browned.

Pot pie with side of mashed potatoes
780 CALORIES
Turkey Mock-Pie
420 CALORIES

You Save **360** CALORIES

Roasted Salmon with Squash

Moist and flavorful, this no-fuss fish doesn't need much enhancement—or complicated cooking. Just pop it in the oven for 15 minutes for a feed-'em-fast supper.

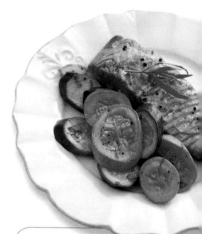

Active time 15 minutes
Total time 30 minutes
Makes 4 servings

- 1 **lemon**
- 4 **pieces (6 ounces each) skinless salmon fillet**
- ½ **teaspoon salt**
- ¼ **teaspoon ground black pepper**
- 4 **medium (8 ounces each) summer squash (zucchini and yellow), each cut diagonally into ½-inch-thick slices**
- 1 **tablespoon chopped fresh tarragon leaves, plus additional sprigs for garnish**

1. Preheat oven to 400°F. From lemon, grate ½ teaspoon peel and squeeze 3 tablespoons juice.

2. Place salmon in 13" by 9" glass or ceramic baking dish. Sprinkle with lemon peel, 1 tablespoon lemon juice, ¼ teaspoon salt, and ⅛ teaspoon pepper. Roast salmon 14 to 16 minutes or until just opaque throughout.

3. Meanwhile, in 4-quart saucepan, place steamer basket over *1 inch water*. Heat water to boiling on high. Add squash; cover and reduce heat to medium. Steam 8 minutes or until tender. Transfer to medium bowl and toss with chopped tarragon, ¼ teaspoon salt, ⅛ teaspoon pepper, and remaining 2 tablespoons lemon juice. Arrange squash and salmon on dinner plates; garnish salmon with tarragon sprigs.

EACH SERVING: ABOUT 275 CALORIES, 37 G PROTEIN, 8 G CARBOHYDRATE, 11 G TOTAL FAT (2 G SATURATED), 93 MG CHOLESTEROL, 375 MG SODIUM, 3 G FIBER

Sample More Seafood

Follow a low-cal diet that includes more fish, and chances are you'll drop more pounds than you would eating the same meal plan minus the seafood, suggests a study published in the *International Journal of Obesity*. One possible explanation: Ounce for ounce, fish has fewer calories than almost all cuts of beef, pork, and skin-on poultry. Researchers theorize that omega-3 fatty acids, the polyunsaturated fats abundant in cold-water fish like salmon and mackerel, switch on the fat-burning process in cells—provided you also exercise.

HEALTHY RECIPE MAKEOVER

New England Clam Chowder

To slim this dish—by more than half the calories and cholesterol of the original—we cut back on the bacon, swapped reduced-fat milk for cream, and stirred in flour in place of several starchy potatoes.

Active time 20 minutes
Total time 50 minutes
Makes 6 servings

- 1½ **cups water**
- 12 **large cherrystone or chowder clams, scrubbed**
- 2 **slices bacon, chopped**
- 1 **medium onion, chopped**
- 1 **medium carrot, chopped**
- 1 **stalk celery, chopped**
- 2 **tablespoons flour**
- 1 **large potato, peeled and cut into ½-inch chunks**
- 2 **cups reduced-fat (2%) milk**
- ⅛ **teaspoon ground black pepper**
- 1 **tablespoon snipped fresh chives**

1. In 4-quart saucepan, heat water to boiling on high. Add clams; return to boil. Reduce heat to medium-low; cover and simmer 10 minutes or until clams open. Discard any unopened clams.

2. Strain clam broth through sieve lined with paper towel into 4-cup liquid measuring cup. Add water to broth to equal 2½ cups total.

3. Rinse saucepan to remove any grit. In same saucepan, cook bacon on medium until browned. With slotted spoon, transfer bacon to plate lined with paper towels to drain. To bacon fat in pan, add onion, carrot, and celery; cook 9 to 10 minutes or until tender, stirring occasionally.

4. Meanwhile, remove clams from shells and coarsely chop. Stir flour into vegetable mixture; cook 1 minute, stirring. Gradually stir in clam broth. Add potato; heat to boiling. Cover; simmer on low 12 minutes or until potato is tender, stirring occasionally. Stir in milk, clams, pepper, and bacon; heat through (do not boil). Sprinkle with chives to serve.

EACH SERVING: ABOUT 180 CALORIES, 8 G PROTEIN, 20 G CARBOHYDRATE, 9 G TOTAL FAT (4 G SATURATED), 21 MG CHOLESTEROL, 155 MG SODIUM, 2 G FIBER

Classic New England clam chowder
SINGLE SERVING: 370 CALORIES
Healthy Makeover New England Clam Chowder
SINGLE SERVING: 180 CALORIES

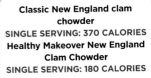

You Save
190
CALORIES

Make It a Drop 5 Meal

Serve with a whole-grain roll (around 100 calories) spread with 1 teaspoon trans-fat-free margarine, as well as 2 cups mixed greens with ½ cup grape tomatoes, 1 tablespoon chopped pecans, and 100-calorie portion of dressing.
COMPLETE MEAL: 482 CALORIES

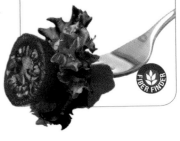

Shepherd's Pie

If you spent your days chasing sheep, maybe—just maybe—you could wolf down the classic version of this dish and stay slim. But the ground lamb alone contains more than three and a half times the fat of our whole casserole. This scrumptious renovation—rich in protein, fiber, and six types of vegetables—trims the calories by more than 50 percent per serving.

Active time 50 minutes
Total time 1 hour 15 minutes
Makes 6 main-dish servings

- 2 **pounds all-purpose potatoes, peeled and cut into quarters**
- ½ **cup low-fat (1%) milk**
- 2 **tablespoons reduced-fat or Neufchâtel cream cheese**
- ¾ **teaspoon salt**
- ¾ **teaspoon ground black pepper**
- 1 **pound extra-lean (97%) ground beef**
- 2 **large onions (10 to 12 ounces each), finely chopped**
- 2 **large carrots, finely chopped**
- 2 **large celery stalks, finely chopped**
- ½ **cup dry white wine**
- 1½ **teaspoons fresh thyme leaves, chopped**
- 1 **package (10 ounces) frozen peas, thawed**
- 1 **package (10 ounces) frozen corn, thawed**

1. In covered 4-quart saucepan, place potatoes and enough cold water to cover; heat to boiling on high. Reduce heat to medium; uncover and simmer 18 minutes or until tender. Drain well; return to saucepan. Add milk, cream cheese, and ¼ teaspoon each salt and pepper; mash until smooth.

2. Preheat oven to 425°F. Heat 12-inch skillet on medium-high until hot. Add beef and ¼ teaspoon each salt and pepper; cook 3 to 5 minutes or until browned and cooked through, stirring. With slotted spoon, transfer beef to large bowl.

3. To same skillet on medium-high, add onions, carrots, celery, and ¼ teaspoon each salt and freshly ground black pepper. Cook 8 minutes or until tender, stirring. Add wine to skillet; cook 2 minutes, stirring to incorporate browned bits from pan, or until

reduced by half. Stir in thyme and beef, along with any juices.

4. In 3-quart shallow baking dish, spread half of potatoes in an even layer. Top with beef mixture, peas, and corn. Spoon remaining potatoes evenly on top; spread to cover filling. Bake 25 minutes or until top is golden brown.

EACH SERVING: ABOUT 350 CALORIES, 25 G PROTEIN, 55 G CARBOHYDRATE, 5 G TOTAL FAT (2 G SATURATED), 44 MG CHOLESTEROL, 360 MG SODIUM, 8 G FIBER

Classic shepherd's pie
SINGLE SERVING: 730 CALORIES
Healthy Makeover Shepherd's Pie
SINGLE SERVING: 350 CALORIES

You Save
380
CALORIES

Make It a Drop 5 Meal
Serve with a whole-grain roll spread with 1 teaspoon trans-fat-free margarine.
COMPLETE MEAL: 478 CALORIES

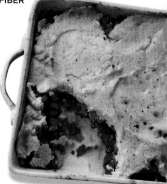

SATISFYING
sweets

We all crave sweets, but they are famous for derailing weight-loss efforts. Whether you like them smooth and creamy, warm or chilly, here are satisfying options that allow you to indulge.

TOP 5 QUICK-FIX TREATS

With the exception of the granita, these are a tad over 100 calories, but you can compensate by adjusting your calorie intake later—or earlier!—in the day.

1. **BALSAMIC BERRIES** Toss 1 cup sliced strawberries with ½ tablespoon melted margarine to coat. Stir in a splash of balsamic vinegar and a pinch of coarsely ground black pepper. **110 CALORIES**

2. **PEACHES AND CREAM** Slice 1 small peach. Sprinkle with cinnamon and microwave for about 30 seconds, until warm. Serve with ½ cup nonfat vanilla frozen yogurt. **133 CALORIES**

3. **PB PUDDING** Warm 1 teaspoon peanut butter in the microwave for 20 seconds on Medium. Stir into 1 container nonfat chocolate pudding. **131 CALORIES**

4. **COFFEE GRANITA** In medium bowl, stir ⅔ cup sugar and 2 cups hot espresso until sugar has completely dissolved. Pour into 9-inch square metal baking pan; cool. Cover, freeze about 2 hours, stir with a fork to break up chunks. Cover and freeze until the mixture is completely frozen, at least 3 hours or overnight. To serve, let the granita stand at room temperature for about 15 minutes. Use a metal spoon to scrape across the surface of the granita, transferring the ice shards to dessert dishes. Top ½ cup granita with 2 tablespoons whipped cream. Makes about 10 servings. **69 CALORIES PER SERVING**

5. **CHOCOLATE FIGS** Slice 2 ripe figs. Melt 2 teaspoons chocolate chips and drizzle over figs. **120 CALORIES**

Strawberry Ice Cream

This delectable four-ingredient treat whips up in 10 minutes flat and freezes into scoopable sweetness in an hour. A serving of labor-intensive, custard-based strawberry ice cream has 282 calories, 12 grams of saturated fat, and 134 times the cholesterol of our luscious dessert, which has a mere 70 calories per serving and less than ½ gram of saturated fat.

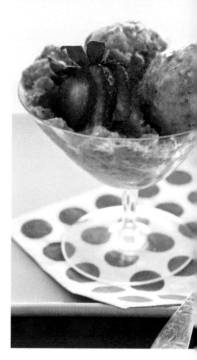

Active time 10 minutes
Total time 10 minutes plus freezing
Makes 3 ½ cups or 7 servings

- **16 ounces frozen strawberries**
- **1 cup 2% plain Greek yogurt (see Tip)**
- **¼ cup sugar**
- **½ teaspoon vanilla extract**
- **Fresh strawberries, sliced, for garnish**

1. In food processor with knife blade attached, pulse 1 cup frozen strawberries until finely chopped. Transfer chopped berries to large metal bowl.

2. In food processor, puree yogurt, sugar, vanilla, and remaining strawberries until smooth. Transfer to bowl with frozen strawberries; stir until well combined. Cover and freeze about 1 hour, until firm but not hard. Garnish with fresh strawberries.

TIP The Greek yogurt provides an especially creamy texture, but if you like, you can swap in low-fat yogurt to further reduce your calories and fat.

EACH ½-CUP SERVING: ABOUT 70 CALORIES, 3 G PROTEIN, 14 G CARBOHYDRATE, 1 G TOTAL FAT (0.4 G SATURATED FAT), 1 MG CHOLESTEROL, 10 MG SODIUM, 1 G FIBER

Classic strawberry ice cream
SINGLE SERVING: 282 CALORIES
Healthy Makeover Strawberry Ice Cream
SINGLE SERVING: 70 CALORIES

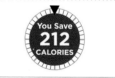

You Save
212
CALORIES

HEALTHY RECIPE MAKEOVER

Chocolate Chip Cookies

Classic chocolate chip cookies
SINGLE SERVING: 160 CALORIES
Healthy Makeover Chocolate Chip Cookies
SINGLE SERVING: 80 CALORIES

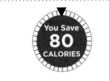

You Save
80
CALORIES

Revamped, these gems are still ooey-gooey good—but they're only 80 calories each (with a gram of healthy fiber per cookie). Lose the guilt—and indulge.

Active time 15 minutes
Total time 27 minutes
Makes 48 cookies

- ½ cup (packed) brown sugar
- ½ cup granulated sugar
- ½ cup trans-fat-free vegetable oil spread (60% to 70% oil)
- 1 large egg
- 1 large egg white
- 2 teaspoons vanilla extract
- 1¼ cups all-purpose flour
- 1 teaspoon baking soda
- ½ teaspoon salt
- 2½ cups quick-cooking or old-fashioned oats, uncooked
- 1 cup bittersweet (62% cacao) or semisweet chocolate chips

1. Preheat oven to 350°F.

2. In large bowl, with mixer on medium-low speed, beat sugars and vegetable spread until well blended, occasionally scraping bowl with rubber spatula. Add egg, egg white, and vanilla; beat until smooth. Beat in flour, baking soda, and salt until mixed.

3. With wooden spoon, stir in oats and chocolate chips until well combined. Drop dough by rounded measuring tablespoons, 2 inches apart, on ungreased large cookie sheet. Bake 12 to 13 minutes or until golden. With wide metal spatula, transfer cookies to wire rack to cool. Repeat until all batter is used.

EACH COOKIE: ABOUT 80 CALORIES, 1 G PROTEIN, 11 G CARBOHYDRATE, 4 G TOTAL FAT (1 G SATURATED), 4 MG CHOLESTEROL, 70 MG SODIUM, 1 G FIBER

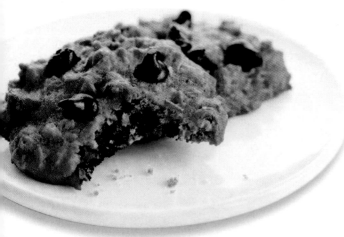

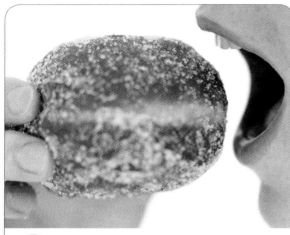

Emotional Eating 101

Overeating can be a way of coping with stress and other emotionally charged situations. And, like other obsessions, you can conquer it. Here's how:

- **Figure out what triggers your eating.** Do you stuff yourself when you are sad, lonely, angry, bored, guilt-ridden? Whatever your triggers, an important part of breaking the emotional eating habit is finding out what's pushing you to turn to food.

- **Eliminate stressors** where possible and think of ways to add more fun and joy to your life.

- **Start using other (healthy!) means to cope.** When you recognize an urge to eat, ask yourself if you are really, truly hungry. Physical hunger tends to be gradual, while an emotional appetite usually comes on suddenly. Brainstorm some activities you could do instead of eating that actually deal with the emotion (meditate, call a friend, write in a journal, etc.), and test them out until you find a few that stick.

Learn from the "Losers"

"Whenever I am tempted to dip into the cookie jar, I take a moment to run through recent triumphs in my head. This positive replay always keeps me on track."

—JESSICA CHICAS,
52 POUNDS LOST

BEFORE

AFTER

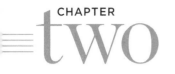

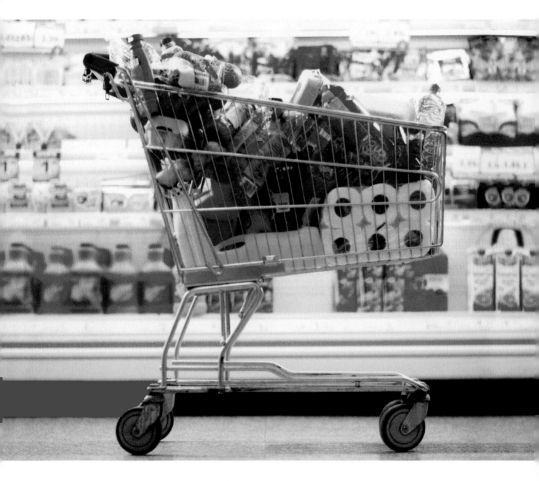

SUPERMARKET SAVVY
shopping for
diet-friendly
foods

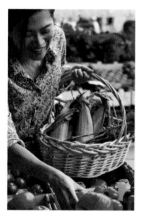

Take the guesswork out of healthy grocery shopping by filling your cart with our weight-busting picks.

GROCERY SHOPPING with your waistline in mind requires a sharp eye. What with some food manufacturers' sneaky marketing tactics, genius product placement, and delicious-smelling sample carts, it's easy to sabotage your diet. And since the average shopper makes two trips to the grocery store per week, that's two times to be tempted.

But these food-buying expeditions don't have to be a giant diet trap. We'll show you how to fill your kitchen with the best choices your store has to offer. We've done the homework for you, scouting out the tastiest brand-name foods—from salad dressings to cheeses to frozen treats, and more—that all fit within the Drop 5 calorie guidelines. Plus, our tips will help you go beyond what we've suggested to create your own list of favorite foods.

Turn the page to see the Drop 5 Top 5 things to consider when you're wheeling your cart down the aisles.

Drop
5 Top 5

SUPERMARKET SAVVY TIPS

1 STICK WITH A LIST Who would have thought that shopping with a carefully crafted grocery list could cut the amount of calories you load into your cart by almost half? In a Lincoln University study, participants who were taught to prepare a weekly menu, convert it into a shopping list, adjust the list for foods already on hand, and organize it according to a supermarket's layout purchased about 6,500 fewer calories per week when compared to their previous trips without the menu and list-making training. That savings, over the remaining seven weeks of the twelve-week study, culminated in a total caloric savings of nearly 46,000 fewer calories. Better still, fewer calories in the cart translated into weight loss—to the tune of at least five pounds per person over the twelve weeks.

What's key is to structure your list around a weekly menu. Set aside time before you shop to plan meals and snacks, taking into consideration your family's competing schedules and what you already have on hand. Use our recipes (see recipe index, page 32), Drop 5 meals, and our Drop 5 three-day sample meal plan (page 20) to help you create a healthy, low-cal menu and shopping list.

Shopping list

☐ Eggs
☐ Milk
☐ Bread
☐ Fruit
☐ Salad greens

Arming yourself with a shopping list will help you avoid high-fat sweets and other impulse purchases. Structure your list around your weekly menu and don't deviate from it.

2 **FAMILY MATTERS** You'll find it much easier to Drop 5 lbs (and keep them off) if you *and* your family adopt a healthier lifestyle. However, when possible, it's best to grocery shop alone. Not only will it speed up your trip, you'll also avoid caving on your kids' and spouse's food demands. But when shopping solo is not an option, find fun ways to involve your family. Plan the week's meals and shopping list together, and then tackle the store as a team. Teach your kids how to read labels (page 24) and encourage them to pick out new fruits, veggies, and other foods for the cart.

Don't worry; you and the family can still include some yummy indulgences! Think moderation instead of elimination, buy in calorie-controlled portions (or divvy up large bags of goodies into smaller packages when you get home), and limit treats to one per person, per trip.

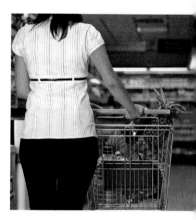

Don't go to the grocery store hungry. Eat a healthy, satisfying meal or small, filling snack first.

3 **EAT BEFORE YOU GO** When you're hungry, every pie, tart, and bag of chips is tantalizing. A full stomach helps you ignore their overtures. If you have to head to the store after work and don't have time to stop and eat before you go, grab a small, filling snack at the store like a string cheese, piece of fruit, or a high-fiber bar.

4 **HANG OUT ON THE EDGE** The bulk of your cart should be stacked with items from the outer aisles of the grocery store: produce, meats, and dairy. Store layouts vary, but the fresh foods are almost always on the perimeter, and the packaged goods in the center. Head to the middle aisles first for things like canned beans, whole-grain cereals, and pastas—but resist going up and down all the center aisles. Linger in the outer aisles instead, where you can pick up perishables after the packaged goods. That way they'll stay fresher and they're less likely to be crushed.

DIET TRAP
Avoiding
New Foods

Your mother was right about this one: You'll never know if you like something unless you sample it. But you not only have to try it, you also have to keep an open mind about it. For most people, losing weight means replacing old habits and calorie-laden foods with new, healthier ones. Challenge yourself to choose one unfamiliar, diet-friendly food on each visit to the grocery store. Pick up some broccolini (a cross between broccoli and Chinese kale), a package of quinoa (a nutty-tasting whole grain), or a container of nonfat Greek-style yogurt on your next shopping trip.

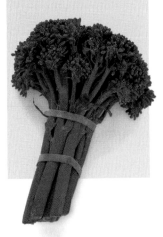

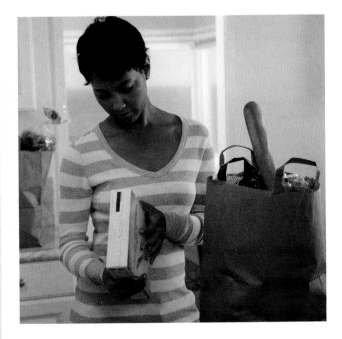

5 BE A LABEL SPY Just because a food is marked nonfat, sugar-free, low-fat, or low-carb doesn't mean it's low in calories, so be sure to carefully read the Nutrition Facts panel. Don't forget to check the serving size, too: Sometimes an item looks like a single serving (a personal-size frozen pizza, a snack-size package of chips or cookies, or an individual beverage bottle), but the nutrition information on the packaging reveals that it's actually two or three servings. That means it's two or three times the calories, fat, sugar, and everything else. (See "Label Lesson" on page 24.)

To save time at the store, or to investigate a product without kids in tow, try reading about products online. Most food companies post full nutrition facts and ingredient lists on their websites, making it a cinch to get informed before you hit the aisles.

DAILY CALORIE TARGETS

Consult these guidelines as you choose
recipes, meals, and snacks from this chapter.

FOR WOMEN		FOR MEN	
Breakfast	350	Breakfast	450
Lunch	500	Lunch	600
Dinner	500	Dinner	600
Snack	100	Snack	200
Optional Treat	100	Optional Treat	200
TOTAL	1,450–1,550	Total	1,850–2,050

If you go a little over (or under) at any meal, compensate by adjusting your calories later in the day. Have the optional treat once a day, or save up those calories and have a larger treat every other day, or even two larger 350-calorie treats a couple of days a week. If you want to cut calories a bit more, you can also skip the optional treat altogether.

Power Shop Online

If you (or your children) just can't seem to resist tossing temptations into your cart, try ordering your groceries online. Researchers in a multi-university study assigned 28 people to either a standard weight-loss program or a program with grocery delivery. After eight weeks, online buyers had fewer fattening products and less total food in their cupboards. Their shopping secret? Virtual grocery carts make it easier to stick to a list—eliminating last-minute cookie grabs. Check your local stores for online shopping options, or try national services like AmazonFresh.com, MyWebGrocer.com, or Netgrocer.com, which deliver all over the country. You'll not only save yourself from the consequences of diet-unfriendly impulse purchases, but you'll also keep a little more cash in your pocket because you're not blowing it on unnecessary extras.

canned & dry goods

From healthy canned or boxed soups to Drop 5 meals featuring canned tuna and salmon, we help you select top-shelf products.

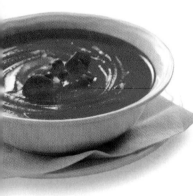

HEALTHY CANNED OR BOXED SOUPS

Ladle these Drop 5 options into your soup bowl.

1. **AMY'S ORGANIC BLACK BEAN VEGETABLE SOUP** 140 CALORIES PER CUP

2. **IMAGINE ORGANIC CREAMY BUTTERNUT SQUASH SOUP** 90 CALORIES PER CUP

3. **PROGRESSO VEGETABLE ITALIANO SOUP** 100 CALORIES PER CUP

4. **HEALTHY CHOICE GARDEN VEGETABLE SOUP** 130 CALORIES PER CUP

5. **CAMPBELL'S SELECT HARVEST GARDEN RECIPES MINESTRONE SOUP** 100 CALORIES PER CUP

LOOK FOR soups with no more than 150 calories and 2 grams of saturated fat per cup. Consider vacuum-sealed, aseptic boxes, which are nestled next to the cans in the store. This innovative packaging requires less processing, so food often retains more taste, color, and texture than what's found in cans.

TOP 5 MEAL IDEAS FOR CANNED FISH

For an even easier packaged fish, check out the no-fuss, no-draining-required variety in vacuum-packed pouches.

1. **SALMON AND BLACK BEAN TORTILLA SALAD** Combine 3 ounces canned, drained pink salmon with 1 chopped garlic clove, 1 tablespoon lime juice, and ¼ teaspoon ground cumin. Stir in ⅔ cup black beans. Spoon mixture over 3 cups mixed greens. Top with 2 tablespoons salsa mixed with 2 tablespoons nonfat sour cream and 1 ounce (17 chips) crushed baked tortilla chips. **514 TOTAL CALORIES**

2. **TUNA ENGLISH MUFFINS** Combine 6 ounces drained tuna packed in water with 2 tablespoons dried cranberries, 1 tablespoon chopped walnuts, ¼ cup chopped celery, 2 teaspoons light mayonnaise, and 1 teaspoon Dijon mustard. Serve open-faced on a toasted whole-grain English muffin topped with 2 lettuce leaves. Serve with 2 cups mixed greens, ½ cup grape tomatoes, and ½ cup sliced cucumbers tossed with 10 to 15 pumps spray dressing. **440 TOTAL CALORIES**

3. **TUSCAN TUNA SALAD** Mash ¼ cup drained canned cannellini beans. Stir in 1 tablespoon chopped fresh basil leaves, 1 teaspoon capers, 2 teaspoons fresh lemon juice, 1 teaspoon olive oil, and 3 ounces drained canned tuna packed in water. Mix in 1 cup arugula. Add salt and pepper to taste. Serve tuna in one 6-inch whole-wheat pita with 1 cup grapes on the side. **498 TOTAL CALORIES**

4. **PASTA WITH TUNA PUTTANESCA** Cook 3 ounces whole-wheat pasta according to package directions, reserve ¼ cup pasta cooking water, and drain. Toss pasta with 2 teaspoons finely chopped shallots, 1 teaspoon capers, 1 teaspoon red wine vinegar, ½ teaspoon olive oil, 3 ounces drained canned tuna packed in water, 1 cup fresh spinach, 1 tablespoon chopped fresh basil leaves, and salt and pepper to taste. **474 TOTAL CALORIES**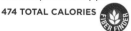

5. **SALMON CAKES** Combine 7 ounces drained canned red or pink salmon, 1 sliced green onion, 4 teaspoons bottled white horseradish, 1 tablespoon plain dried bread crumbs, ½ teaspoon soy sauce, and a few grinds of black pepper. Shape mixture into two 3-inch patties. In nonstick skillet coated with cooking spray, cook salmon cakes over medium heat until golden and heated through, about 5 minutes per side. Serve with 8 spears steamed asparagus and 1 ounce pita chips. **505 TOTAL CALORIES**

Cut Back on Sugar

The average American consumes 22 teaspoons of added sugar (sugars and syrups that are added to foods during processing or preparation, including those added at the table) per day—that's a disaster if you're trying to Drop 5. Sugar adds empty calories and little nutrition to your diet, so it's a good idea to cut back on the sweet stuff, in all its forms. Trouble is, it's lurking in products you'd never suspect.

Most package labels list sugar content in grams—there are roughly 4 grams (or 16 calories' worth) of sugar in a teaspoon. Be aware that the total sugar content on a label doesn't always mean *added* sugar. The natural sugars in foods and drinks like yogurt and juice are also included in the count. Take the Nutrition Facts labels shown below. You might be tempted to pick the product on the left and save 6 grams of sugar. But that label comes from cherry Kool-Aid, and its 16 grams of sugar are all added, so you get calories but not natural nutrients. The label on the right is for Tropicana Pure Premium orange juice, and its 22 grams of sugar are a natural component of the orange, part of a healthy package that includes a variety of vitamins, minerals, and phytochemicals (plant nutrients).

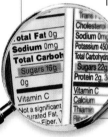

To decode this information when you're grocery shopping, check out the ingredient list on the package. Steer clear of products that list sugar among the first three ingredients. And be on the lookout for the sweetener's many aliases, including these -ose words—glucose, fructose, sucrose, lactose, and maltose—as well as syrup (such as high-fructose corn syrup or brown rice syrup), evaporated cane juice, cane crystals, fruit juice concentrate (such as grape or white grape), honey, and molasses. In the end, they all spell sugar.

Drop

5 DO IT NOW Look for Unsweetened Choices

It's easy to **pick up** a jar of applesauce, pasta sauce, or peanut butter without realizing that a lot of sugar has been added. One leading **pasta sauce**, for instance, has 24.4 teaspoons of sugar in a 26-ounce jar, while a similar sauce from another manufacturer has **only 2.5 teaspoons.** For foods like these, which often taste great without sweeteners, be sure to check the **ingredient list** and look for unsweetened or only slightly sweetened alternatives.

SHOPPING FOR
snacks & drinks

Choosing healthy snacks and beverages on the fly can be a challenge. Our tips will help you make low-cal choices that'll keep you going—and energized.

HEALTHY CONVENIENCE SNACKS

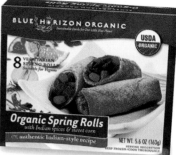

These delicious treats deliver satisfaction at around 100 calories each.

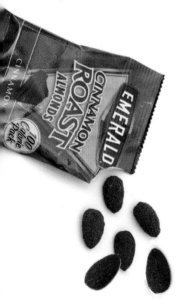

1. **BLUE HORIZON ORGANIC INDIAN-STYLE SPRING ROLLS** Down a few for a spicy snack. **110 CALORIES PER 3 ROLLS**

2. **FIBER ONE 90-CALORIE CHOCOLATE CHEWY BAR** Filled with fiber and delicious. **90 CALORIES PER BAR**

3. **QUAKER CHEWY CHOCOLATE CHIP GRANOLA BARS** Twenty-five percent less sugar and fewer calories equal better Drop 5 snacking. **100 CALORIES PER BAR**

4. **FIG NEWTONS 100% WHOLE GRAIN** The cookie you know from childhood has gotten a whole-grain makeover. **110 CALORIES PER 2 COOKIES**

5. **EMERALD WALNUTS AND ALMONDS 100-CALORIE PACKS** Satisfy snack attacks—and get your vitamin E and healthy omega-3 fats at the same time. **100 CALORIES PER PACKAGE**

Drop 5

DO IT NOW Snack Smarter Your twice daily 100-calorie Drop 5 snacks can be **indulgent treats** (cookies, chips) or a healthy way to **stave off hunger** (fruit, vegetables, yogurt, nuts, whole-grain snacks) until your next meal. If your **favorite treat** does not come in 100-calorie prepackaged servings, divide it into 100-calorie portions yourself.

snacks & drinks

BEFORE YOU DRINK, THINK!

Americans drink 22 percent of their daily calories, according to a recent study. All calorie counts below are for 12-ounce servings. Of course, refreshing, zero-calorie water is your best Drop 5 beverage choice.

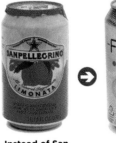

Instead of San Pellegrino Limonata...

...try Fresca

DIET MADNESS	DIET MAKEOVER	YOU SAVE	SWAP ONCE A DAY
Newman's Own Orange Mango Tango 225 CALORIES	Honest Ade Orange Mango with Mangosteen 72 CALORIES	**153** CALORIES	Drop 1 lb in just over **3** WEEKS
Coca-Cola 150 CALORIES	Diet Coke 0 CALORIES	**150** CALORIES	Drop 1 lb in **3½** WEEKS
San Pellegrino Limonata 150 CALORIES	Fresca 0 CALORIES	**150** CALORIES	Drop 1 lb in **3½** WEEKS
IZZE Sparkling Grapefruit 102 CALORIES	Hint Mango-Grapefruit 0 CALORIES	**102** CALORIES	Drop 1 lb in **5** WEEKS

Calorie-Burning Drinks

On the shelves Enviga, Celsius, Fuze Healthy Infuzions Slenderize, Skinny Water beverages, JavaFit Diet Plus coffees

Claims Slogans include "The great taste of burning calories!" and "Lose weight—gain energy." Some of the products promise to curb appetite, boost your metabolism, and burn fat.

Evidence The key ingredient in many of these beverages is green tea extract or caffeine or, often, a combination of the two. Short-term studies have shown that these additions can give your metabolism a small boost (about 3.5 percent in one study of the combo) and burn an average of 78 calories. But in a 2006 issue of *Obesity Reviews,* researchers noted that additional studies were needed to determine whether the products actually help you lose in the real world, over the long haul. Some products include ingredients that you often find in over-the-counter weight-loss supplements, including *Citrus aurantium* (bitter orange), *chromium picolinate,* or *Garcinia cambogia* (a type of fruit native to India). But in a recent article in *Obesity Management*, George Bray, MD, of the Pennington Biomedical Research Center, concluded there was little to no evidence that these ingredients make it easier to drop pounds.

Shopping bottom line These products are calorie free (or virtually so). If you have a sugary-soda habit, switching to any diet drink can help you lose. Just don't count on the "calorie-burning" additives in these beverages to make a huge difference.

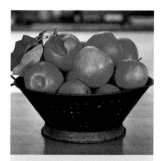

MAKE IT A HABIT
Buy Whole Fruits Rather than Fruit Juices

You'll feel fuller on fewer calories and get more healthy fiber from the actual fruit. A cup of apple juice, for example, has no fiber and more than 100 calories, but a cup of sliced apple (about one small apple) has 74 calories and more than 3 grams of fiber.

SHOPPING FOR
grains

Whole-grain foods can help you Drop 5 because they contain more fiber and are more filling, which leaves you feeling satisfied. Bonus: They have more healthy nutrients. To get the most bang for your buck, look for products that are 100 percent whole grain. (See the "Eat More Fiber Index," page 258, for a list of recipes containing 5 grams of fiber or more.)

Get the Whole-Grain Truth

If the label does not say "100% whole grain," check the ingredient list for refined culprits.

FIRST

It's a Whole Grain If It's Called:

- Brown rice
- Buckwheat
- Bulgur or cracked wheat
- Millet
- Quinoa
- Sorghum
- Triticale
- Wheat berries
- Whole-grain barley or pearled barley
- Whole-grain corn
- Whole oats or oatmeal
- Whole rice
- Whole rye
- Whole spelt
- Whole wheat

It's *Not* a Whole Grain If It's Called:

- Corn flour
- Cornmeal
- Degerminated cornmeal
- Enriched flour
- Pumpernickel
- Rice
- Rice flour
- Rye flour or rye
- Stone-ground wheat (if whole grain, label should say "stone-ground whole wheat")
- Unbleached wheat flour
- Wheat
- Wheat flour
- Wheat germ (it's not a whole grain, but wheat germ is still good for you)

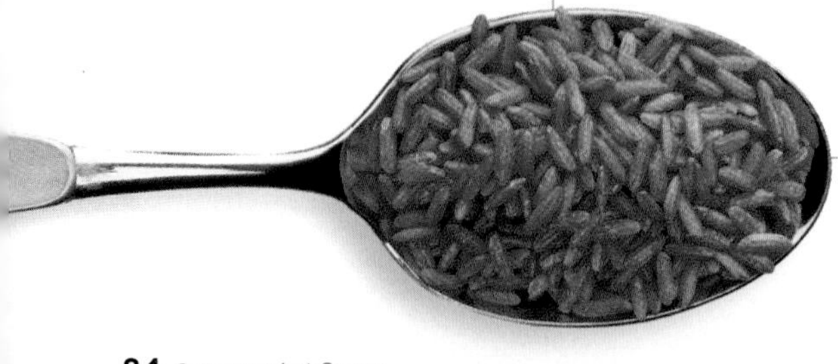

HEALTHY CONVENIENCE GRAIN DISHES

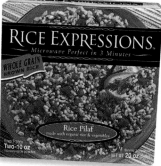

1. **RICE-A-RONI SPANISH WHOLE GRAINS BLENDS** A spicy side dish with whole-grain brown rice, tomatoes, onions, and peppers. **250 CALORIES PER CUP**

2. **RICE EXPRESSIONS WHOLE GRAIN BROWN RICE PILAF** Its ingredient list is short and sweet: organic brown rice and veggies. **166 CALORIES PER CUP**

3. **SEEDS OF CHANGE DHARAMSALA INDIAN RICE BLEND** An aromatic blend of rice, beans, potatoes, vegetables, and spices. **210 CALORIES PER CUP**

4. **KASHI 7 WHOLE GRAIN ORIGINAL PILAF SEVEN WHOLE GRAINS AND SESAME** offers nutrient-dense calories and lots of fiber. **340 CALORIES PER CUP**

5. **SEEDS OF CHANGE TIGRIS MIXTURE OF SEVEN WHOLE GRAINS** The essential goodness of ancient grains that's on your table in just 90 seconds. **270 CALORIES PER CUP**

LOOK FOR 100 percent whole-grain pasta, rice, and more with no more than 1 gram of saturated fat and at least 3 grams of fiber per ½ cup (dry) serving.

Picking Pasta

Opt for 100 percent whole-grain pasta. Keep in mind that some whole-grain pastas are chewier and grittier and some shapes taste better than others. There are plenty to choose from, so if at first you don't succeed, try (another brand), try (another shape—say, linguine if you didn't like the spaghetti) again. Or, since some whole grain is better than none at all, choose multigrain pasta, which is better than white pasta.

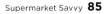

HEALTHY CEREALS

Fill your cereal bowl with these tasty options.

1. MULTIGRAIN CHEERIOS

110 CALORIES PER CUP

2. KELLOGG'S RAISIN BRAN

190 CALORIES PER CUP

3. KASHI HEART TO HEART HONEY TOASTED OATS

120 CALORIES PER ¾ CUP

4. GENERAL MILLS WHEAT CHEX

160 CALORIES PER ¾ CUP

5. QUAKER LOWER SUGAR INSTANT OATMEAL MAPLE & BROWN SUGAR

120 CALORIES PER PACKET

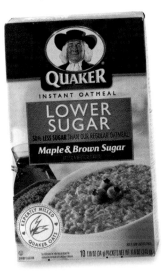

LOOK FOR cereals that list bran, wheat germ, or a whole grain (like oats or whole wheat), before sugar in the ingredients list. Cereals should also have at least 3 grams of fiber per serving (about 1 cup for cold cereal or ½ cup, uncooked, for hot cereal) and the less sugar the better. Note: If a cereal includes real fruit—for example, Raisin Bran—there's no sugar limit because there is naturally occurring sugar in fruit.

Drop

5 DO IT NOW Add Fruit to Your Cereal Adding fresh **sliced berries,** bananas, peaches, or whatever is **in season** to your bowl of whole-grain cereal is a wonderful way to sneak more fruit into your diet. It not only **adds sweet flavor,** it also provides lots of **satisfying fiber.**

HEALTHY CRACKERS

Opt for these good-for-you whole-grain snacks.

1. **AK-MAK STONE GROUND WHOLE WHEAT SESAME CRACKERS**
   115 CALORIES PER 5 CRACKERS

2. **KASHI HEART TO HEART WHOLE GRAIN ROASTED GARLIC CRACKERS**
   120 CALORIES PER 7 CRACKERS

3. **WASA ORIGINAL WHOLEGRAIN CRISPBREAD** **80 CALORIES PER 2 SLICES**

4. **TRISCUIT ROSEMARY AND OLIVE OIL CRACKERS** **120 CALORIES PER 5 CRACKERS**

5. **WHEAT THINS 100% WHOLE GRAIN CRACKERS** **140 CALORIES PER 16 CRACKERS**

LOOK FOR 100 percent whole-grain crackers with no more than 140 calories and 1 gram saturated fat (no trans fat) per 1-ounce (28-gram) serving.

HEALTHY BREAD

Grainy bread is one of the most satisfying foods around.

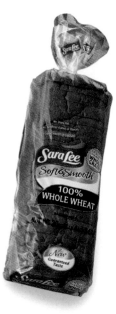

1. **FLATOUT HEALTHY GRAIN MULTI-GRAIN WRAP**
   100 CALORIES PER FLATBREAD

2. **THOMAS' BETTER START LIGHT MULTI-GRAIN ENGLISH MUFFIN**
   100 CALORIES PER MUFFIN

3. **PEPPERIDGE FARM 100% NATURAL 100% WHOLE WHEAT BREAD**
   100 CALORIES PER SLICE

4. **SARA LEE SOFT & SMOOTH 100% WHOLE WHEAT BREAD**
   75 CALORIES PER SLICE

5. **WONDER STONEGROUND 100% WHOLE WHEAT BREAD**
   90 CALORIES PER SLICE

LOOK FOR 100 percent whole-grain bread, tortillas, pitas, buns, or flatbread with at least 2 or 3 grams fiber and no more than 100 calories per slice or serving.

SHOPPING FOR
produce

Our "Healthiest Fruits and Vegetables" steer you toward the most nutrient-packed produce. Our picks are packed with vitamins, minerals, and phytochemicals— health-boosting plant compounds— including lycopene (found in watermelon and grapefruit), lutein (in greens and broccoli), carotenoids (in sweet potatoes, papaya, and butternut squash), and more!

HEALTHIEST FRUITS

FRUIT SERVING	CALORIES	FIBER	OTHER GOOD THINGS
½ grapefruit (pink or red)	52	2 g	Pink and red varieties have more antioxidants and phytochemicals than their white or yellow cousins
1 whole kiwifruit	42	2 g	Ounce for ounce, kiwis contain more vitamin C than an orange. Also loaded with vitamin K, folate, and potassium
1 cup cubed papaya	55	2½ g	Rich in vitamins A and C and potassium. The seeds are also delicious and nutritious
1 cup halved strawberries	49	3 g	Packed with vitamin C, folate, fiber, and flavor
1 cup cubed watermelon	46	½ g	Has more lycopene than any other fruit or vegetable. Also rich in vitamins A and C

HEALTHIEST VEGETABLES

VEGETABLE SERVING	CALORIES	FIBER	OTHER GOOD THINGS
1 cup chopped broccoli	30	2½ g	Rich in vitamins K and C, carotenoids, calcium, iron, and potassium
1 cup Brussels sprouts	33	3 g	Contains vitamins K and C, and carotenoids, calcium, iron, and potassium
2 cups raw greens such as spinach, kale, and collards	14	1½ g	Rich in vitamins A, C, and K, as well as folate, potassium, magnesium, iron, lutein, and other phytochemicals
1 cup cubed butternut squash	63	3 g	Loaded with potassium, magnesium, and vitamins A and C
1 (5-inch) sweet potato	112	4 g	Packed with carotenoids, vitamin C, potassium, and fiber

produce

MAKE IT A HABIT
Add Fresh Vegetables or Fruit to Your Frozen Meals

To create a satisfying 500-calorie Drop 5 lunch or dinner, supplement your frozen pizza, entrée, or sandwich with a side of fresh vegetables or fruit, a salad, or a frozen veggie side dish like Birds Eye Steamfresh or Green Giant Simply Steam. You'll not only fill up on the fiber, you'll also boost your intake of vitamins and minerals.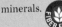

Buy Preprepped Produce

With already peeled, cut, and washed fruit and veggies on hand, you'll be less likely to turn to unhealthy choices. While they cost more than whole produce, they're hassle-free and time-saving.

- **PREWASHED SALAD GREENS** It's easy to eat salads more often when all you have to do is dump and dress. Look for darker greens and mixed greens, which pack more nutrition per bite (see Meal Ideas for Prewashed Bagged Spinach, opposite).

- **PRECUT FRUIT** If you're counting on fruit to help you through a sweet craving, it's got to be ready when the need strikes. Be sure to purchase packages without added sugar. Precut fruit can also reduce the chance that you'll buy a whole fruit and forget it in your crisper.

- **PRECUT SLAW** Talk about versatility in a bag. Look for plain, precut veggie slaw (sans the fatty dressing, of course) and try it sautéed with a little oil for a quick side dish, mix it with veggies for a stir-fry, or use it to bulk up homemade or canned soups.

Stop the Cart for Spinach!

Spinach nutritionally outscores even the much-praised broccoli with its long list of vitamins and minerals. This leafy wonder is also one of the richest sources of lutein, a plant chemical that protects against age-related blindness. It's convenient, too: Just open a bag of prewashed spinach for salads or sandwiches. Or pop it right in the microwave for two to three minutes for a convenient side dish. To economize, cook a package of frozen spinach, which is just as nutritious.

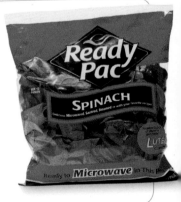

TOP 5 MEAL IDEAS FOR PREWASHED BAGGED SPINACH

1. **SPINACH SCRAMBLE** In nonstick skillet coated with cooking spray, sauté ½ red pepper, chopped, until tender. Add 1 cup spinach and cook until just wilted, about 1 minute. Stir in 2 beaten eggs and 2 tablespoons crumbled feta cheese and cook, stirring frequently, until eggs are firm and cooked through. Serve with 1 slice whole-wheat toast spread with 2 teaspoons trans-fat-free margarine. **343 TOTAL CALORIES**

2. **SPINACH SALAD WITH CHICKEN** Combine 3 cups spinach with ½ cup sliced cucumber, ½ cup cherry tomatoes, ¼ cup dried cranberries, and 2 tablespoons low-fat, reduced-calorie balsamic vinaigrette. Top with 3 ounces chopped, cooked skinless chicken breast (can be sliced from a rotisserie chicken) and 1 ounce crumbled goat cheese. Serve with 1 whole-grain roll. **490 TOTAL CALORIES** 🌾FIBER FINDER

3. **SPINACH AND HUMMUS FLATBREAD** In nonstick skillet coated with cooking spray, sauté 1 sliced yellow pepper with 1 cup sliced mushrooms until just tender. Add 1 cup spinach and cook until wilted. Spread a multigrain flatbread (such as Flatout Flatbread) with ½ cup hummus. Top with ¼ cup each sliced cucumbers, sliced or shredded carrots, and crumbled feta; add spinach mixture, and roll up. **468 TOTAL CALORIES** 🌾FIBER FINDER

4. **SPINACH AND WHITE BEAN PASTA** Sauté 2 cloves chopped garlic in ½ tablespoon olive oil. Stir in ¼ cup canned white beans (navy, cannellini, or Great Northern, rinsed and drained). Cook, stirring occasionally, until heated through. Spoon onto 1 cup cooked multigrain pasta and toss with 2 cups spinach, stirring until wilted. Top with 1 tablespoon grated Parmesan cheese. Serve with salad: 2 cups mixed greens and ½ cup grape tomatoes tossed with 10 to 15 pumps spray dressing. **495 TOTAL CALORIES** 🌾FIBER FINDER

5. **SPINACH AND TORTELLINI** In a nonstick skillet coated with cooking spray, sauté 2 chopped garlic cloves, 1 large sliced portobello mushroom, ¾ cup halved cherry tomatoes, and ½ cup thawed frozen peas until mushrooms are tender, about 5 minutes. Add 2 cups spinach and sauté until wilted, 1 to 2 minutes. Remove from heat and toss with 1 cup cooked fresh cheese tortellini; top with 3 tablespoons grated Parmesan cheese and 1 tablespoon pine nuts. Season with salt and pepper. Serve with 2 cups mixed greens tossed with 10 to 15 pumps spray dressing. **460 TOTAL CALORIES** 🌾FIBER FINDER

produce

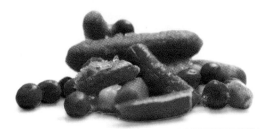

TOP 5 MEAL IDEAS FOR FROZEN VEGETABLES

1. **BROCCOLI-CHEDDAR SCRAMBLE** Scramble 2 eggs with ½ cup thawed, frozen broccoli florets. Just before eggs are cooked, top with 1 tablespoon shredded low-fat cheddar cheese. Add salt and pepper to taste. Serve with 1 slice whole-wheat toast topped with 1 teaspoon trans-fat-free margarine, and ½ cup grapes. **341 TOTAL CALORIES**

2. **OPEN-FACED MEXICAN VEGGIE BURRITO** Place an 8-inch flour tortilla on a microwave-safe plate. Top the tortilla with ½ cup canned refried beans, ¼ cup shredded low-fat cheddar cheese, ¼ cup diced avocado, and ½ cup frozen corn. Roll burrito and microwave for 30 seconds or until heated through. Serve with ¼ cup prepared salsa.
474 TOTAL CALORIES

3. **SHRIMP RICE WITH BABY PEAS** Sauté 4 ounces shrimp in 1 teaspoon olive oil. When shrimp are almost cooked through (about 3 minutes), add 2 tablespoons white wine or chicken broth and 1 cup thawed frozen baby peas. Cook until peas are heated through. Pour shrimp and pea mixture over 1 cup cooked whole-wheat linguine; toss with 2 tablespoons shredded Parmesan cheese. Top with 1 tablespoon chopped fresh parsley and season with salt and pepper to taste. **466 TOTAL CALORIES**

4. **PASTA SALAD WITH CHICKEN AND MIXED VEGGIES** Combine 3 ounces cubed, cooked skinless chicken breast, ½ cup thawed frozen mixed vegetables, 1½ cups chopped cherry tomatoes, and ¼ cup garbanzo beans with 1 cup cooked whole-wheat rotini. Toss with 1 teaspoon olive oil, 1 teaspoon red wine vinegar, and salt and pepper to taste. **497 TOTAL CALORIES**

5. **SNOW PEA STIR-FRY** Cut 3 ounces pork tenderloin into bite-sized pieces. Heat a wok over high heat, add 1 teaspoon peanut oil, then add pork. Cook until pork browns, then remove from wok. Add 1 teaspoon peanut oil to wok and cook 2 teaspoons minced garlic, 2 teaspoons minced ginger, and 1 cup thawed frozen snow peas until peas soften and begin to brown, then add pork back to wok with ½ teaspoon soy sauce and 1 to 2 teaspoons lime juice. Serve over 1 cup brown rice. **447 TOTAL CALORIES**

MYTH BUSTER

Fiction Frozen fruits and vegetables are less nutritious than fresh ones. **Fact** That's true only if you live on a farm. Produce picked at the peak of ripeness does have more vitamins and minerals, but nutrient levels drop during shipping and storage. And they sink even further if you add the days that the produce lingers in your crisper. Frozen veggies and fruit, on the other hand, are usually picked ripe and immediately flash frozen, so they retain most of their nutrients. For calorie control, be sure to select frozen produce without added sugar, syrup, sauce, or cheese.

Stop the Cart for Pears!

Thanks to a corrected calculation by the U.S. Food and Drug Administration, we now know pears are even higher in fiber. At 6 grams (formerly 4 grams) per medium-size pear, they're a great, filling food—perfect for slicing into salads or enjoying as a sweet, healthy dessert.

CRAVING 911

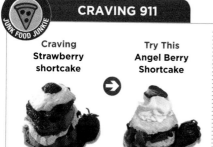

Craving	Try This
Strawberry shortcake	Angel Berry Shortcake

Take a 1-ounce piece of angel food cake (see page 241) and cut it into 2 thin slices. Place slices from 2 strawberries between the pieces. Top with ¼ cup light whipped topping and 1 additional sliced strawberry.

Strawberry shortcake
420 CALORIES
Angel Berry Shortcake
125 CALORIES

You Save
295
CALORIES

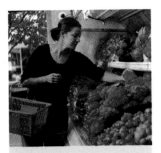

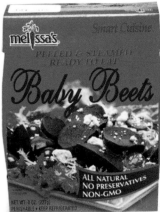

DIET TRAP
Not Eating Enough Produce

Researchers at Pennsylvania State University randomly assigned 97 obese women to two groups. One group was counseled to simply reduce their fat intake, while the other was told to lower the fat and eat more water-rich foods, particularly fruit and vegetables. After one year, all the women had lost weight, but the second group had dropped 3.3 more pounds on average, with a total average loss of 17 pounds.

The difference: Produce-aisle foods are fiber-packed and filling and they're also low-cal. Plus, the second group focused on what they could eat as opposed to what they needed to avoid.

HEALTHY CONVENIENCE FRUITS AND VEGGIES

These time-saving products are ready to eat or need only be reheated in the microwave.

1. **MELISSA'S PEELED & STEAMED READY TO EAT BABY BEETS** Naturally rich in potassium—toss 'em in salads or sandwiches. **40 CALORIES PER 2½ BEETS**

2. **SIMPLY POTATOES MASHED SWEET POTATOES** These savory potatoes are sweetened with brown sugar and cinnamon. **90 CALORIES PER ½ CUP**

3. **CEDAR'S CHICKPEA SALAD** A mouth-watering medley of garbanzo beans, veggies, and dried cranberries. **160 CALORIES PER ½ CUP**

4. **JUST FRUIT MUNCHIES** Crunchy, delicious bits of freeze-dried fruit available in packs of apples, raisins, blueberries, sour cherries, mango, pineapple, and raspberries. **100 CALORIES PER 1 OUNCE**

5. **MELISSA'S STEAMED READY TO EAT LENTILS** Ladle these tasty legumes into soups and salads. **115 CALORIES PER ½ CUP**

HEALTHY SALAD DRESSINGS

There's nothing like salad dressing to load up on the fat and calories. Happily, these healthy dressings are low in both.

1. **ANNIE'S NATURALS LITE HONEY MUSTARD VINAIGRETTE** 40 CALORIES PER 2 TABLESPOONS

2. **KEN'S STEAK HOUSE FAT FREE RASPBERRY PECAN** 50 CALORIES PER 2 TABLESPOONS

3. **NATURALLY FRESH LITE PEPPERCORN RANCH** 80 CALORIES PER 2 TABLESPOONS

4. **NEWMAN'S OWN LIGHTEN UP BALSAMIC VINAIGRETTE** 45 CALORIES PER 2 TABLESPOONS

5. **WISH-BONE SALAD SPRITZERS CAESAR DELIGHT** 10 CALORIES PER 10 SPRAYS

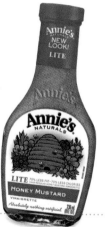

LOOK FOR salad dressings with no more than 100 calories and 2 grams of saturated fat per 2 tablespoons. Opt for pump or spray dressings, and you'll get around 10 calories per 10 pumps—plenty to coat a plate of greens.

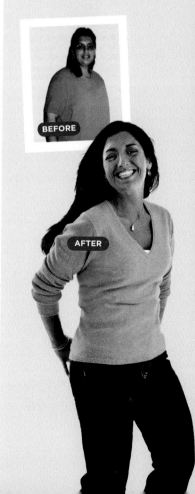

SHOPPING FOR
meat, poultry & seafood

Need help navigating your way around the meat counter? Our shopping tips and recipes—including five ideas for Drop 5 dinners based on rotisserie chicken and flank steak—will lead the way. And don't forget to incorporate good-for-your-heart fatty fish, or the low-calorie protein power of tofu.

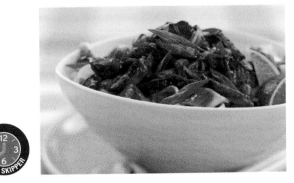

HEALTHY CONVENIENCE MEATS AND POULTRY

Low-cal dinners are easy to prepare with these convenient products.

1. **GOURMET DINING PORK STIR FRY** Restaurant flavor without the extra calories or artery-clogging fat.
   190 CALORIES PER 8 OUNCES

2. **HORMEL TURKEY MEAT LOAF** Hearty and nutritious comfort food that's ready in just minutes.
   190 CALORIES PER 5 OUNCES

3. **LAURA'S LEAN BEEF SHREDDED BEEF WITH BARBECUE SAUCE** This hormone-free beef is bathed in a tangy BBQ sauce. **245 CALORIES PER 5 OUNCES**

4. **GOURMET DINING GARLIC CHICKEN SKILLET MEAL** Garlic fans will be thrilled with this simple skillet dish.
   210 CALORIES PER 8 OUNCES

5. **LAURA'S LEAN BEEF POT ROAST AU JUS** This crowd-pleaser tastes like it's been slow-cooked for hours.
   110 CALORIES PER 3 OUNCES

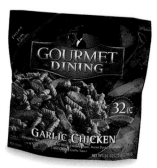

CHOOSE CALORIE-CONSCIOUS CUTS

(per 6 ounces cooked meat, off the bone and sauce-free)

Instead of pork ribs...　　　**...try pork tenderloin**

DIET MADNESS	DIET MAKEOVER	YOU SAVE	SWAP TWICE A WEEK
Pork ribs **558 CALORIES**	Pork tenderloin **250 CALORIES**	**308** CALORIES	Drop 1 lb in **5½** WEEKS
Prime rib **480 CALORIES**	Beef tenderloin **240 CALORIES**	**240** CALORIES	Drop 1 lb in **7** WEEKS
70% lean ground beef **464 CALORIES**	95% lean ground beef **291 CALORIES**	**173** CALORIES	Drop 1 lb in **10** WEEKS
Chicken leg with skin **394 CALORIES**	Chicken breast without skin **280 CALORIES**	**114** CALORIES	Drop 1 lb in **15** WEEKS

meat, poultry & seafood

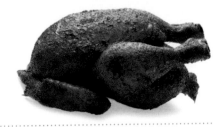

🌿 TOP 5 MEAL IDEAS FOR ROTISSERIE CHICKEN

1. **WALDORF SALAD** Combine 1½ cups broccoli slaw (such as Mann's), 1 cup chopped or shredded skinless, boneless white breast meat (or ¾ cup dark meat) from a rotisserie chicken, 1 cup chopped Granny Smith apple (about 1 small), ¼ cup halved seedless grapes, 1 tablespoon chopped walnuts, and 1 tablespoon crumbled blue cheese. Stir in 3 tablespoons plain nonfat yogurt, 1 tablespoon lemon juice, and ⅛ teaspoon ground black pepper. Serve over 2 cups mixed greens. **470 TOTAL CALORIES**

2. **CARIBBEAN WRAP** Combine ½ cup chopped or shredded skinless, boneless white breast meat (or ⅓ cup dark meat) from a rotisserie chicken with 2 tablespoons chopped red onion, 2 chopped garlic cloves, ½ cup cubed mango, ¼ cup drained and rinsed low-sodium black beans, a pinch of red pepper flakes, and 2 teaspoons chopped cilantro. Spoon into a whole-wheat tortilla and roll up. Serve with 2 tablespoons roasted macadamia nuts and 2 cups mixed greens tossed with 10 to 15 pumps spray dressing. **485 TOTAL CALORIES**

3. **MEDITERRANEAN COUSCOUS** Combine ¾ cup cooked whole-wheat couscous with ½ cup rinsed and drained low-sodium cannellini beans, ¼ cup chopped red onion, ½ cup halved grape tomatoes, ¼ cup marinated artichoke hearts, and ½ cup chopped or shredded skinless, boneless white breast meat (or ⅓ cup dark meat) from a rotisserie chicken. Drizzle with 3 tablespoons lemon juice, 1 teaspoon olive oil, 2 tablespoons chopped fresh basil, and 2 tablespoons crumbled feta cheese. Season with ground black pepper and a sprinkle of sea salt. Serve with a plum or tangerine. **520 TOTAL CALORIES**

4. **CHICKEN AND ARTICHOKE PASTA** In a skillet coated with cooking spray, combine ½ cup chopped marinated artichoke hearts, ¼ cup chopped tomatoes, 1 tablespoon chopped Kalamata olives, and 1 cup chopped skinless, boneless white breast meat (or ¾ cup dark meat) from a rotisserie chicken and cook until warmed through. Serve over 1 cup cooked whole-grain penne and top with 1 tablespoon feta cheese and 2 tablespoons chopped basil. Season with ground black pepper and a sprinkle of salt. **515 TOTAL CALORIES**

5. **OPEN-FACED CHICKEN QUESADILLA** Place one 8-inch whole-wheat tortilla in a medium skillet coated with cooking spray. Top with ¾ cup shredded skinless, boneless white breast meat (or ⅔ cup dark meat) from a rotisserie chicken, 6 tablespoons reduced-fat shredded cheddar cheese, and 2 tablespoons chopped green onions. Cook until the bottom tortilla browns and cheese melts, about 5 minutes. Serve with ¼ cup salsa and 2 cups mixed salad greens with 100 calories dressing. **479 TOTAL CALORIES**

Surprising Good-for-Your-Waist Picks

BEEF TENDERLOIN STEAKS Ounce for ounce, this melt-in-your-mouth cut has about the same calorie and fat content as skinless chicken thighs.

CHICKEN THIGHS They are higher in fat and calories than breasts, but as long as you remove the skin and any excess fat, economical thighs fit into a good-for-you diet. They also provide 25 percent more iron and more than twice as much zinc as the same amount of breast meat.

PORK Tenderloin and boneless loin chops compare favorably, calorie wise, with skinless chicken. So, if your family is crying "fowl," vary the menu with these lean, healthy cuts of pork.

Stop the Cart for Fatty Fish!

Omega-3 fats are good for your heart, but they can also be a boon to your waistline. In a multicenter study involving 232 overweight volunteers on a reduced-calorie diet, researchers found that when the dieters ate a meal rich in fatty fish, they felt fuller longer than those who had eaten a leaner fish, such as cod.

The reason? High levels of omega-3s may prompt the body to produce more leptin—the hormone that signals fullness. And this may lead you to eat less food throughout the day, scientists hypothesize. One easy way to get these good-for-you fats: Use canned salmon, which is less expensive than fresh.

Stop the Cart for Tofu!

You won't find it in the meat section, but tofu's protein does the job of its meaty cousins. It may seem too light to be filling, but a Louisiana State University study found that tofu is a mighty diet food. Researchers tested it against chicken as an appetizer for 42 overweight women—and the participants who had tofu ate less food during the meal that followed. The secret: Tofu seemed to quash hunger more than chicken.

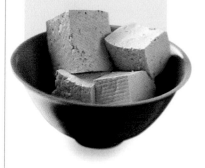

meat, poultry & seafood

Learn from the "Losers"

"I won't go grocery shopping when I'm hungry! If fattening foods aren't in my home, I can't eat them!"

**—KAREN DUSHOK,
109 POUNDS LOST**

"I'm with Oprah—no eating after 7 p.m. I also steer clear of TV; for me, it leads to grazing. Instead, I keep busy—doing chores, writing in my journal, or running."

**—SUSAN HAUGLAND,
100 POUNDS LOST**

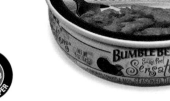

HEALTHY CONVENIENCE SEAFOOD

Select from salmon fillets to crab and shrimp cakes—all ready in a jiffy.

1. **BUMBLE BEE SENSATIONS EASY PEEL BOWL SUNDRIED TOMATO & BASIL** A tasty tuna mix full of heart-healthy omega-3s. **130 CALORIES PER BOWL**

2. **GOURMET DINING SHRIMP STIR FRY** Shrimp, sauce, and enough veggies to provide plenty of vitamins A and C. **200 CALORIES PER 8 OUNCES**

3. **MOREY'S SEASONED GRILL MARINATED WILD ALASKAN SALMON** These individually frozen six-ounce fillets are loaded with omega-3s and perfectly seasoned without too much salt. **270 CALORIES PER 6 OUNCES**

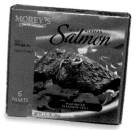

4. **CHICKEN OF THE SEA SMOKED PACIFIC SALMON** Packaged in a ready-to-eat, freshness-preserved pouch, this is an easy, healthy, and tasty meal starter. **120 CALORIES PER POUCH**

5. **PHILLIPS CRAB AND SHRIMP CAKES** You'll love the tongue-tingling spices in this seafood pairing. **170 CALORIES EACH**

TOP 5 MEAL IDEAS FOR FLANK STEAK

Start with cooked flank steak (broil, bake, or sauté with cooking spray until done, about ten minutes), and you can whip up these hearty Drop 5 meals in just ten minutes more.

1. **GREEK STEAK SALAD** Mix 6 ounces cubed cooked flank steak with 2 cups mixed greens, ½ cup each halved cherry tomatoes and chopped cucumber, ¼ cup crumbled feta cheese, 2 tablespoons olives, 2 teaspoons each red wine vinegar and olive oil, and salt and pepper to taste. Serve with one 4-inch whole-wheat pita. **490 TOTAL CALORIES**

2. **STEAK FAJITA WRAPS** Heat one 8-inch whole-wheat tortilla in the microwave for 10 seconds, or until soft. Top tortilla with 3 ounces sliced cooked flank steak, ¼ cup each prepared salsa and sliced avocado, and 2 tablespoons shredded reduced-fat cheddar cheese. Wrap the tortilla around the fillings. Heat in a nonstick skillet, toaster oven, or microwave, or serve cold. Enjoy with a medium apple or pear. **480 TOTAL CALORIES**

3. **STEAK PESTO PASTA** Cook 2 ounces whole-grain penne pasta according to package directions. Drain and mix with 3 ounces cubed cooked flank steak, 2 tablespoons prepared pesto sauce, and 1 cup each baby spinach leaves and chopped tomatoes. For dessert, have 1 cup berries. **510 TOTAL CALORIES**

4. **STEAK FRIED RICE** In medium skillet, heat 1 teaspoon peanut oil over medium-high heat and add ¼ teaspoon each minced garlic and minced ginger and 2 teaspoons chopped green onions; cook for 1 minute. Add 1 cup cooked brown rice and cook 2 to 3 minutes, stirring. Add 3 ounces cubed cooked flank steak and stir in 1 tablespoon soy sauce. Serve with 1 cup steamed snow peas. **446 TOTAL CALORIES**

5. **THAI STEAK NOODLES** Prepare 2 ounces rice noodles according to package directions. Mix with 3 ounces cubed cooked flank steak; 1 teaspoon rice vinegar; 1½ teaspoons peanut oil; 1 teaspoon soy sauce; and ¼ teaspoon each honey and chili garlic sauce (or to taste). Top with 2 sliced green onions and 1 tablespoon roasted peanuts. Serve with 1 cup steamed broccoli. **492 TOTAL CALORIES**

SHOPPING FOR
dairy

Milk, yogurt, eggs, and cheese are all great sources of calcium and protein. In fact, see the Moo-Chew Connection, opposite, to learn how eating more calcium-rich dairy foods may help you lose weight.

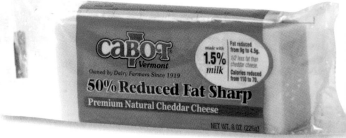

MYTH BUSTER

Fiction Low-fat dairy is not as nutritious as full-fat dairy.

Fact Contrary to popular belief, low-fat dairy products like milk, cheese, and yogurt supply all the vitamins and minerals you'd get from their full-fat cousins. The only things missing are the extra fat and calories.

HEALTHY CHEESES

1. **CABOT 50% REDUCED FAT SHARP CHEDDAR**
   70 CALORIES PER 1-OUNCE SERVING

2. **ORGANIC VALLEY LOW-FAT COTTAGE CHEESE**
   100 CALORIES PER ½ CUP

3. **LAUGHING COW MINI BABYBEL LIGHT**
   50 CALORIES PER PIECE

4. **LAUGHING COW ORIGINAL OR LIGHT CREAMY SWISS** 50 OR 35 CALORIES PER PIECE

5. **SARGENTO LIGHT STRING CHEESE**
   50 CALORIES PER PIECE

LOOK FOR cheese (including hard cheese, string cheese, cream cheese, cheese spreads, and goat cheese) with no more than 70 calories and 3 grams of saturated fat per 1-ounce serving. Cottage cheese (½ cup serving) and ricotta cheese (¼ cup serving) should have no more than 100 calories and 2 grams of saturated fat.

HEALTHY YOGURT

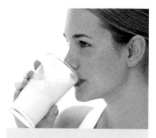

1. DANNON LIGHT-'N-FIT YOGURT (any flavor)

80 CALORIES PER 6-OUNCE SERVING

2. FAGE TOTAL 0% YOGURT (plain)

90 CALORIES PER 6-OUNCE SERVING

3. LA YOGURT BLENDED LOWFAT YOGURT (blueberry)

100 CALORIES PER 6-OUNCE SERVING

4. STONYFIELD FARM OIKOS 0% FAT ORGANIC GREEK YOGURT (any flavor)

80 TO 120 CALORIES PER 5.3-OUNCE SERVING

5. YOPLAIT LIGHT THICK & CREAMY YOGURT (any flavor)

100 CALORIES PER 6-OUNCE SERVING

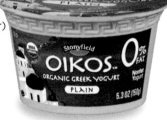

LOOK FOR yogurt with no more than 120 calories and 2 grams of saturated fat per 6-ounce serving.

MAKE IT A HABIT
Switch to 1 Percent or Nonfat Milk

How do you wean yourself from stocking your fridge with whole or 2 percent milk? One step at a time. If you're drinking whole, go to 2 percent for a few weeks, then try 1 percent for a while. You can stop there, or go on to enjoy nonfat (it has 90 calories per cup, about 20 fewer than 1 percent). Also try products like Farmland Dairies Skim Plus or Skinny Cow Fat-Free Milk (110 calories per cup)—they have additional protein and calcium, which gives them a creamy taste without the fat.

The Moo-Chew Connection

Eating more calcium-rich dairy foods may help you Drop 5. Studies have found that adults who eat a calcium-rich, high-dairy diet lose more weight and fat than those who consume a low-dairy diet with the same number of calories. Researchers speculate that calcium-rich dairy foods may boost the body's fat burning after a meal.

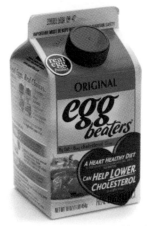

MYTH BUSTER

Fiction The cholesterol in eggs is bad for you.
Fact One large egg has 213 milligrams cholesterol, and health experts suggest limiting dietary cholesterol to 300 milligrams a day or less (200 milligrams a day if you have heart disease, diabetes, or high LDL "bad" cholesterol). However, dietary cholesterol's effect on blood cholesterol is still a mystery, and studies suggest that saturated fat and trans fat may have a much bigger impact.

If you have cardiovascular disease, diabetes, or high LDL cholesterol, you should eat no more than two eggs per week, but you can have as many egg whites as you like (the cholesterol is in the yolk). Try products like Eggology On-the-Go Egg Whites (zap for 95 seconds in the microwave and presto—a scramble filled with 13 grams of hunger-sating protein) and Egg Beaters.

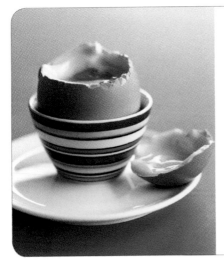

Stop the Cart for Eggs!

When researchers tracked people on a low-cal diet, they found that those who ate two eggs for breakfast lost 65 percent more weight than those who had a bagel—even though they consumed the same number of calories. (Plus, the egg eaters' cholesterol levels didn't go up.) They shed the extra pounds because they felt fuller after breakfast and ate fewer calories throughout the day.

SHOPPING FOR
frozen food

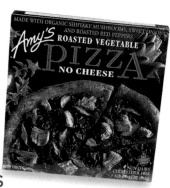

Afraid that the temptations of the frozen food aisles will derail your Drop 5 efforts? Here are our guidelines for frozen dinners, pizzas, ice cream, and more.

LOOK FOR frozen meals, pizzas, and sandwiches with no more than 300 calories and 4 grams of saturated fat (no trans fat), and at least 3 grams of fiber per meal, sandwich, or 6-ounce portion of pizza (about a third of a 10-inch pie). Opt for whole-grain choices whenever you can find them. Round out your meal with veggies or a salad.

HEALTHY FROZEN MEALS AND PIZZAS

1. **AMY'S ROASTED VEGETABLE PIZZA**
   270 CALORIES PER ⅓ PIZZA

2. **HEALTHY CHOICE CAFÉ STEAMERS GRILLED CHICKEN MARINARA** 270 CALORIES PER ENTRÉE

3. **KASHI ALL NATURAL MUSHROOM TRIO & SPINACH THIN CRUST PIZZA** 250 CALORIES PER ⅓ PIZZA

4. **LEAN CUISINE SPA CUISINE LEMONGRASS CHICKEN**
   260 CALORIES PER ENTRÉE

5. **WEIGHT WATCHERS SMART ONES FRUIT INSPIRATIONS CRANBERRY TURKEY MEDALLIONS** 250 CALORIES PER ENTRÉE

HEALTHY FROZEN HEAT-AND-EAT SANDWICHES

1. **AMY'S SPINACH FETA IN A POCKET SANDWICH**
   260 CALORIES PER SANDWICH

2. **AUNT TRUDY'S ROASTED VEGETABLE FILLO POCKET SANDWICH**
   240 CALORIES PER SANDWICH

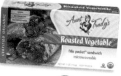

3. **CEDARLANE LOW FAT BEANS, RICE & CHEESE STYLE BURRITO** 260 CALORIES PER SANDWICH

4. **KASHI POCKET BREAD CHICKEN RUSTICO SANDWICH**
   300 CALORIES PER SANDWICH

5. **KASHI POCKET BREAD TURKEY FIESTA SANDWICH**
   270 CALORIES PER SANDWICH

HEALTHY FROZEN DESSERTS

Indulge in these light and creamy options.

1. BREYERS SMOOTH & DREAMY FAT FREE CHOCOLATE FUDGE BROWNIE ICE CREAM 110 CALORIES PER ½ CUP

2. EDY'S SLOW-CHURNED MINT CHOCOLATE CHIP ICE CREAM 120 CALORIES PER ½ CUP

3. SHARON'S RASPBERRY SORBET 100 CALORIES PER ½ CUP

4. SKINNY COW CHOCOLATE TRUFFLE BARS 100 CALORIES PER BAR

5. STONYFIELD FARMS ORGANIC GOTTA HAVE JAVA FROZEN YOGURT 100 CALORIES PER ½ CUP

LOOK FOR low-fat ice cream, frozen yogurt, sorbet, or frozen novelties with no more than 120 calories and 2 grams saturated fat (no trans fat) per ½ cup serving or per bar.

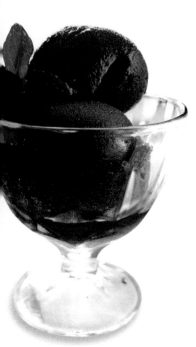

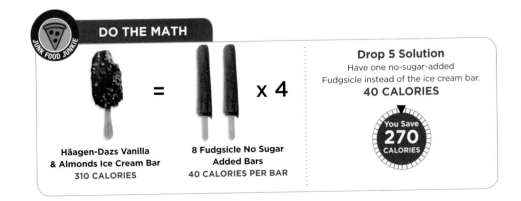

DO THE MATH

= **x 4**

Häagen-Dazs Vanilla & Almonds Ice Cream Bar
310 CALORIES

8 Fudgsicle No Sugar Added Bars
40 CALORIES PER BAR

Drop 5 Solution
Have one no-sugar-added Fudgsicle instead of the ice cream bar.
40 CALORIES

You Save
270
CALORIES

WE ALL SCREAM FOR ICE CREAM

Take note of these luscious Drop 5 swaps.

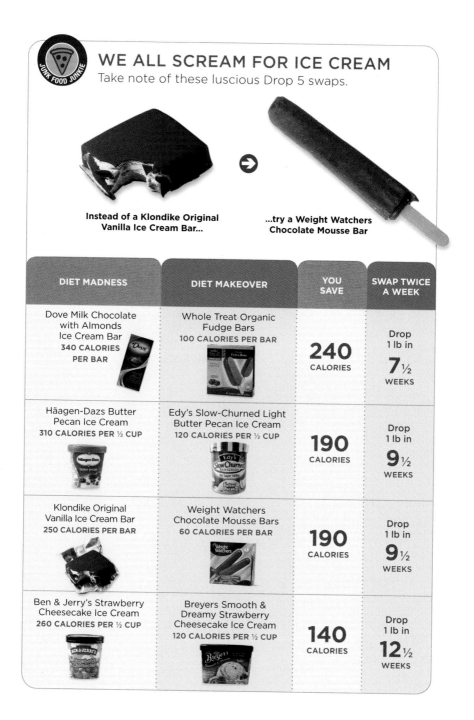

Instead of a Klondike Original Vanilla Ice Cream Bar...

...try a Weight Watchers Chocolate Mousse Bar

DIET MADNESS	DIET MAKEOVER	YOU SAVE	SWAP TWICE A WEEK
Dove Milk Chocolate with Almonds Ice Cream Bar **340 CALORIES PER BAR**	Whole Treat Organic Fudge Bars **100 CALORIES PER BAR**	**240** CALORIES	Drop 1 lb in **7½** WEEKS
Häagen-Dazs Butter Pecan Ice Cream **310 CALORIES PER ½ CUP**	Edy's Slow-Churned Light Butter Pecan Ice Cream **120 CALORIES PER ½ CUP**	**190** CALORIES	Drop 1 lb in **9½** WEEKS
Klondike Original Vanilla Ice Cream Bar **250 CALORIES PER BAR**	Weight Watchers Chocolate Mousse Bars **60 CALORIES PER BAR**	**190** CALORIES	Drop 1 lb in **9½** WEEKS
Ben & Jerry's Strawberry Cheesecake Ice Cream **260 CALORIES PER ½ CUP**	Breyers Smooth & Dreamy Strawberry Cheesecake Ice Cream **120 CALORIES PER ½ CUP**	**140** CALORIES	Drop 1 lb in **12½** WEEKS

ON THE JOB
rules of thumb
to follow
at work

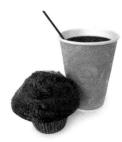

Are you in a mocha-plus-mega-muffin rut? Recognize it and replace this routine with a healthier habit, such as a skim milk latte with low-fat yogurt and fruit.

WHEN YOU START YOUR WORKDAY, you may have the best of intentions. You resolve to eat a wholesome breakfast at home, but you're late so you grab a doughnut from the office café instead. Or you plan on going for a brisk walk at lunch—but then a client calls unexpectedly and you're stuck on the phone during your lunch hour. Or you'd like to turn down a slice of your coworker's birthday cake. But wouldn't it be rude to refuse?

Relax. An occasional slip-up isn't the end of the world—not if you're following the Drop 5 plan. Incorporate these simple strategies into your workday, and you'll be on your way to a slimmer version of you.

Turn the page for our Drop 5 Top 5 tips to make weight loss one of your job's benefits.

Drop 5 Top 5

ON-THE-JOB HOW-TOS

1 **BUDDY UP** Ask your coworkers—there are probably a few of them who also want to Drop 5—to form a weight-loss team. Start an at-work potluck and ask team members to sign up to bring healthy lunch dishes to share on certain days, take walks during coffee breaks or at lunchtime, and exchange low-calorie recipes. Create an e-mail group to track the team's weekly pounds lost, number of minutes exercised, and favorite weight-loss tips.

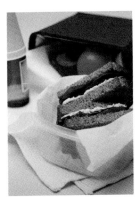

You'll save money and time by brown bagging it. And you'll be less tempted by high-calorie lunch options at the deli near your office.

2 **BROWN BAG IT** Instead of eating lunch out, where you're more likely to give in to calorie-filled choices, whenever possible, bring your lunch to work. Don't think you have time? Try packing something for yourself while you're making your kids' lunches. For grab-and-go lunches the whole week through, keep your freezer stocked with figure-friendly frozen options (see page 105 for suggestions) or portion out dinner leftovers into single serving packages to take to work the next day. If you like to socialize with your coworkers at lunchtime, encourage them to bring their lunches, too. The bonus? You'll save money and time by eating in—and you can use the rest of your lunch hour to take a quick, energizing walk before getting back to work. There will be days, of course, when packing a lunch isn't an option;

you'll be going out for a coworker's birthday, or you have a noontime work meeting. This doesn't mean you have to throw your diet out the window. As often as possible, choose foods that are nutrient-dense for energy (like sandwiches with whole-grain bread and lean deli meat), fiber-packed to curb hunger (like salads, vegetables, and fruits), and calorie-controlled for weight loss. You'll thereby offset any less stellar choices you make and set yourself up for long-term Drop 5 success.

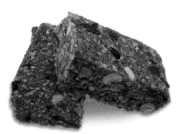

Keep a stash of low-calorie snacks in your purse, desk drawer, locker, or workplace fridge.

3 MIX IT UP Maybe you're in a rut—on your way to work, you always stop at the local coffee shop for a mocha and a pastry, or when three p.m. rolls around, you take a trip to the vending machine for a bag of chips. Recognize your routines and replace them with healthier habits. For example, swap a low-cal nonfat latte for the mocha, and instead of the cheese Danish, try one of the quick and satisfying breakfasts on page 114. Instead of the chips, munch on low-fat microwave popcorn. Remember, even small changes to your rituals can make big changes in your waistline.

4 BUILD A SNACK ARSENAL Snacking not only keeps energy levels up, it also staves off hunger until your next meal. But sometimes it's easy to get caught up in a day's duties and deadlines without refueling. Keep low-cal snacks in your purse, desk drawer, locker, or workplace fridge so you're less likely to sabotage your Drop 5 efforts when you get a snack attack at work. (See "Workplace Snacks to Stash" on page 121.)

DIET TRAP
Keeping Treats in Plain Sight

If you keep sweets and other empty-calorie foods out of sight in your workplace, it'll be much easier to keep them out of mind. Experts at Cornell University determined that women ate more Hershey's Kisses when the candies were on their desks and visible than when they were on their desks in opaque containers.

What to do about the candies on other people's desks and the treats in the break room? Whenever possible, avoid your at-work sweet danger zones (if need be, politely explain to friends why you are no longer visiting their desks), practice portion control (have one candy corn, not twenty), and try keeping sugar-free hard candies or gum in your desk and purse to help control sweet cravings. But the best defense against high-calorie snacking is simply staying full. Fill up on office-friendly Drop 5 breakfasts (page 114), lunches (page 116), and snacks (page 121), and you'll be better prepared to turn down treats.

5 WORK IT OUT Australian researchers examined data on nearly 1,600 male and female full-time office workers. They found that workers sat an average of more than three hours a day, with 25 percent of them sedentary on the job for more than six hours a day. A higher total daily sitting time was associated with a 68 percent increased risk of being overweight or obese. Get physical to compensate for your sedentary workday. Join a gym, take an early-morning run, find time for fitness fun with your family, and use the tips and tricks in this chapter and in Fitness First (page 180) to incorporate more movement into your life.

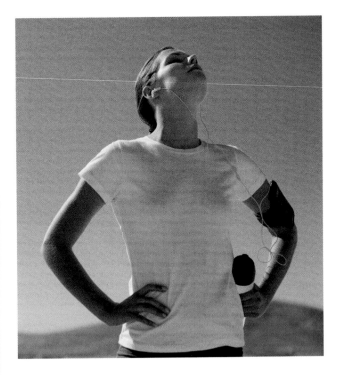

DAILY CALORIE TARGETS

Consult these guidelines as you choose
recipes, meals, and snacks from this chapter.

FOR WOMEN		FOR MEN	
Breakfast	350	Breakfast	450
Lunch	500	Lunch	600
Dinner	500	Dinner	600
Snack	100	Snack	200
Optional Treat	100	Optional Treat	200
TOTAL	1,450–1,550	Total	1,850–2,050

If you go a little over (or under) at any meal, compensate by adjusting your
calories later in the day. Have the optional treat once a day, or save up those
calories and have a larger treat every other day, or even two larger 350-calorie
treats a couple of days a week. If you want to cut calories a bit more, you can
also skip the optional treat altogether.

Drop

5 **DO IT NOW Plan When and Where You'll Eat** "Whether
you **work** in an office or some other setting, it's important
to **plan when** and where you **will eat.** Perhaps you'll go **outdoors**
and sit on a bench for a quick bite or have a mini meal in the
cafeteria. The key is to not let too many **hours pass** before you
eat again, so you're not making a run to the vending machine,"
says nutritionist Elisa Zied, MS, RD, CDN.

breakfasts

Getting the kids ready for school, walking the dog, making yourself presentable for a day at work—there are so many excuses to skip a wholesome breakfast in favor of a fat-loaded pastry or egg sandwich and a latté from a fast-food joint. Our Breakfast Breakdown choices remove the obstacles: These are quick and easy meals to enjoy at home, pack up and eat on the run, or nibble at your desk when you arrive at the office.

Breakfast Breakdown

 To guarantee you never bypass this meal again, here are twelve healthy ways to start your day. Each of these morning options tallies up to roughly 350 calories.

EASY AT-HOME BREAKFASTS

- **BERRY PARFAIT** Combine one 8-ounce container plain low-fat yogurt with 1 cup berries. Drizzle with 1 tablespoon honey and top with ¼ cup low-fat granola-style cereal.

- **CEREAL AND FRUIT** One cup whole grain cereal (like Kashi GoLean) topped with 1 tablespoon sliced almonds, ¼ cup dried apricots (no sugar added), and 1 cup nonfat milk. Or try your cereal dry and enjoy an extra ¼ cup dried apricots.

- **OATMEAL WITH APPLES AND PECANS** Prepare 1 package maple and brown sugar instant oatmeal according to package directions. Stir in ½ tablespoon chopped pecans and 1 small chopped apple (about 1 cup). Pour on 1 cup nonfat milk.

- **FRUIT AND CHEESE** Slice medium apple and top with 1 ounce reduced-fat cheddar cheese (such as Cabot 50% Reduced Fat sharp cheddar); have with ¼ cup almonds.

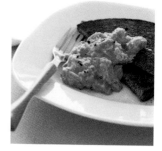

GRAB-AND-GO BREAKFASTS

- **SMOOTHIE** In blender combine ½ cup frozen unsweetened fruit (any variety), ½ cup nonfat milk, ½ cup orange juice, and ⅓ cup dry, unflavored oatmeal. Pour into travel cup.

- **PB AND B** Spread 1 slice whole-grain bread with 1½ tablespoons peanut butter, add slices from ½ banana. Drizzle with 1 teaspoon honey and fold over.

- **EGG ROLLUP** Fill a whole-wheat tortilla with 1 scrambled egg or egg substitute. Microwave 1 slice Canadian bacon about 1 minute on High. Chop, add to tortilla with ½ cup raw baby spinach, and roll up.

- **WAFFLE SANDWICH** Toast 2 frozen waffles, then layer with 1 ounce reduced-fat cheese and 1 slice ham.

ON-THE-JOB BREAKFASTS

- **CAMPER'S DELIGHT** Munch on ¼ cup trail mix (raisins, nuts, sunflower seeds) and sip 1 cup prepared instant hot chocolate.

- **SWEET AND SALTY** Spread 6 reduced-fat Triscuits with 1½ tablespoons almond butter. Have with 1 tangerine or Clementine.

- **BAR BREAKFAST** Pair a Fiber One 90-calorie chewy bar (any flavor) with a banana and 1½ cups vanilla soy milk.

- **CRUNCHY FRUIT CREATION** Stir 1 small handful of almonds (whole or sliced) into a single-serving fruit cup in its own juice.

MYTH BUSTER

Fiction Skipping breakfast will help you lose weight. **Fact** Not eating meals can lead to weight gain. A recent British study that tracked 6,764 people found that breakfast skippers gained twice as much weight over the course of four years as breakfast eaters. Another research group analyzed government data on 4,200 adults. They found that women who ate breakfast tended to eat fewer calories over the course of the day.

WORKDAY LUNCHES
& munchies

Lunch break should be just that—a break. Whether you're brown bagging it, eating at your desk, or going out, here are tips for making your lunch break work for you *and* your waistline. Along the way, we offer advice on healthy snacking the Drop 5 way.

BROWN BAG LUNCHES

1. **TUNA AND CRACKERS** Spoon a 5-ounce package StarKist Tuna Creations (any flavor) onto 10 Triscuits. Pair with 1 cup baby carrots and 1 small fruit, such as a nectarine or a kiwifruit. **505 TOTAL CALORIES**

2. **SOUP LUNCH** Warm 1 can bean or bean-and-vegetable soup and serve with 1 whole-grain roll and 1 cup grapes. **490 TOTAL CALORIES**

3. **SIMPLE SANDWICH** Toast 2 slices whole-wheat bread. Spread one piece with 2 teaspoons grainy mustard and the other with 1 tablespoon low-fat mayonnaise. Layer with 5 slices deli turkey, 4 thin slices green apple, 1 ounce thinly sliced reduced-fat cheddar, and 2 pieces red leaf lettuce. Serve with 1 tangerine. **465 TOTAL CALORIES**

4. **HUMMUS AND VEGGIES** Have ½ cup store-bought hummus with 1 ounce (about 17 chips) baked corn chips, and 1 cup each sliced cucumber, red peppers, and carrots. **480 TOTAL CALORIES**

5. **FROZEN MEAL** Prepare frozen entrée of your choice (with around 300 calories and at least 3 grams of fiber) according to package directions. Serve with 2 cups mixed greens and 1 cup grape tomatoes tossed with 10 to 15 pumps spray vinaigrette and 1 orange for dessert. **480 TOTAL CALORIES**

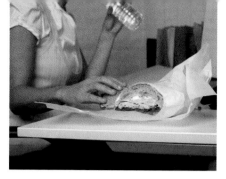

Desktop Dining

Eating at your office desk doesn't have to be off limits, but it can be risky business. Here's what to keep in mind:

PROS "If eating at your desk allows you to have a healthy lunch and means you end up with enough time to take a walk, then it can work in your favor," says Karen Collins, MS, RD, CDN, nutrition advisor to the American Institute for Cancer Research.

CONS "Your desk is a minefield of distractions, so chances are you'll be multitasking while eating—this can not only leave you unsatisfied, but you're also likely to eat past fullness, since mindless eating is a recipe for overeating," says Elisa Zied, author of *Nutrition at Your Fingertips*.

BOTTOM LINE The best meals are the ones that get your undivided attention. If work is front and center, enjoying a good lunch is not. If you must dine at your desk, be sure to stop working and concentrate on eating.

MAKE IT A HABIT
Don't Eat What You Don't Really Want

Why waste calories on banana bread brought in by a coworker if it's not a favorite treat? You can always say, "I'm not hungry right now." Or if politeness dictates that you take a slice, say that you're saving it for later. And make sure to toss it out discreetly at your first opportunity.

Drop

5 **DO IT NOW Be Proactive** If your workplace cafeteria doesn't offer **healthy** choices, find out who's in charge of the **food service,** and lobby for better picks. Ask your supervisor to arrange for health professionals (nutritionists, fitness experts, and the like) to speak to employees over an informational lunch. Start a **walking group** at work. Take personal responsibility for your weight-loss goals and help make your workplace as healthy as possible.

TEST YOUR OUT-TO-LUNCH
CALORIE IQ

Heading out for lunch? See if you can identify the lower-calorie dishes.

Bottom line: It's difficult to spot menu items that are Drop 5 friendly just by their names. Healthy-sounding dishes are often loaded with fat and calories.

WHICH HAS MORE CALORIES...

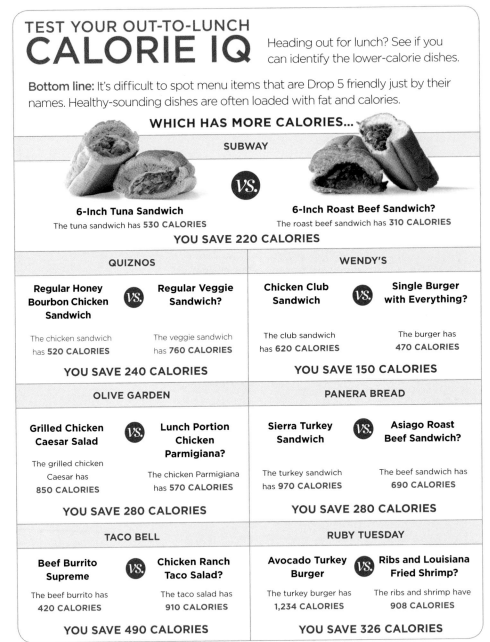

SUBWAY

6-Inch Tuna Sandwich vs. **6-Inch Roast Beef Sandwich?**

The tuna sandwich has **530 CALORIES**   The roast beef sandwich has **310 CALORIES**

YOU SAVE 220 CALORIES

QUIZNOS

Regular Honey Bourbon Chicken Sandwich vs. **Regular Veggie Sandwich?**

The chicken sandwich has **520 CALORIES**   The veggie sandwich has **760 CALORIES**

YOU SAVE 240 CALORIES

WENDY'S

Chicken Club Sandwich vs. **Single Burger with Everything?**

The club sandwich has **620 CALORIES**   The burger has **470 CALORIES**

YOU SAVE 150 CALORIES

OLIVE GARDEN

Grilled Chicken Caesar Salad vs. **Lunch Portion Chicken Parmigiana?**

The grilled chicken Caesar has **850 CALORIES**   The chicken Parmigiana has **570 CALORIES**

YOU SAVE 280 CALORIES

PANERA BREAD

Sierra Turkey Sandwich vs. **Asiago Roast Beef Sandwich?**

The turkey sandwich has **970 CALORIES**   The beef sandwich has **690 CALORIES**

YOU SAVE 280 CALORIES

TACO BELL

Beef Burrito Supreme vs. **Chicken Ranch Taco Salad?**

The beef burrito has **420 CALORIES**   The taco salad has **910 CALORIES**

YOU SAVE 490 CALORIES

RUBY TUESDAY

Avocado Turkey Burger vs. **Ribs and Louisiana Fried Shrimp?**

The turkey burger has **1,234 CALORIES**   The ribs and shrimp have **908 CALORIES**

YOU SAVE 326 CALORIES

MYTH BUSTER

Fiction Eating the day's foods in certain combinations will help you slim down. **Fact** Seventy years ago, Good Housekeeping Research Institute experts declared this fad nonsense, and we say the same thing today. Almost all foods are combinations of protein, fat, and carbohydrates. In whole milk, for instance, about 20 percent of the calories are from protein, 50 percent from fat, and 30 percent from carbohydrates. The digestive system has no problem handling different types of food at the same time. If you do happen to shed pounds on a "food-combining" diet, it's simply because you're eating fewer calories overall.

Savor Meal Memories

To curb late-afternoon snack attacks, think about lunch. In a recent study, British researchers fed 47 women a midday meal and then, three hours later, asked them to write about either the meal or their morning commute. Those who described lunch downed one-third fewer goodies later in the day than those who recalled their travel routine. Why? Remembering your last meal helps activate your body's natural "I'm satisfied" signal, say researchers, so you eat less overall.

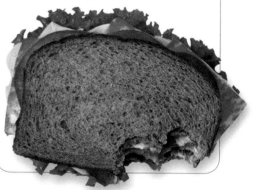

DO THE MATH

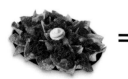 **=** 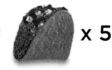 **x 5**

1 Taco Bell Nachos Bellgrande
770 CALORIES

5 Taco Bell Fresco Crunchy Tacos
150 CALORIES EACH

Drop 5 Solution
Have one crunchy taco instead of the nachos.
150 CALORIES

You Save **620** CALORIES

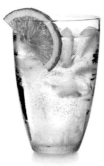

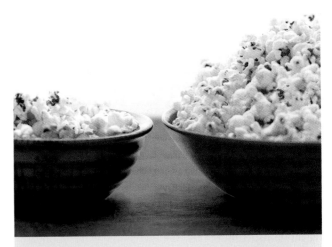

DIET TRAP
Mistaking
Thirst for Hunger

That afternoon stomach pang or feeling of fatigue may be your body's way of asking for a glass of water, not a bag of vending-machine chips. How can you tell? When you feel the urge to eat, start by drinking a cup or two of H_2O (or another zero-calorie drink like club soda, diet soda, seltzer, or unsweetened tea) and see how you feel in five minutes.

Is Popcorn Always a Healthy At-Work Snack?

Nope. Even within the same brand, there can be a big calorie difference in microwave popcorns.

3	**=**	**9**
CUPS		CUPS
Orville Redenbacher's Pour Over Movie Theater Butter Popcorn		**Orville Redenbacher's Smart Pop Butter Popcorn**

Drop 5 Solution
Try individual 100-calorie packs of popcorn.

Vending Machine Know-How

If you know that occasionally you'll fall victim to the lure of the vending machine (almost no one's immune), make your picks ahead of time so your choices are waistline friendly. Scan the offerings and then do some investigating—look up calories and ingredients online or read the nutrition facts labels in grocery stores. Then select items with the lowest number of calories and the most nutrition. And remember, the more filling fiber a food has, the better. Nuts, whole-grain granola bars, trail mix, or whole-grain crackers or pretzels are all good picks.

WORKPLACE SNACKS TO STASH

Snacks in 100-calorie portions are convenient for tossing in your bag as you run out the door. But some are healthier than others. These ten are all smart choices. (Note: Some need to be stored in a freezer or fridge.)

Campbell's Soup at Hand Vegetable with Mini Round Noodles Portable, delicious, and chock-full of veggies.

South Beach Living Snack Bar Delights All five flavors (chocolate mint, chocolate raspberry, whipped chocolate almond, whipped berry, and peanut butter) are loaded with fiber and calcium. They also provide protein, nine vitamins, and minerals.

Blue Bunny FrozFruit Chunky Strawberry Bars High in vitamin C and flavor.

Fudgsicle 100-Calorie Bars These chocolate pops are a source of calcium and snack satisfaction.

Mott's Original Apple Sauce Single-Serving Cups While a fresh apple gives you more fiber, this cup of applesauce also counts as a serving of fruit.

Earthbound Farm Carrot Dippers with Organic Ranch Dip Fresh veggies (and only a bit of dip).

Yoplait Smoothie Light Provides protein and fiber; it's also an excellent source of calcium.

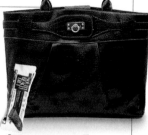

Sun Chips 100 Calorie Mini Bites Snack Packs This multigrain snack packs 5 grams of fiber and supplies hard-to-find vitamin E.

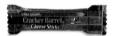

Cracker Barrel 2% Milk Cheese Sticks The fat is a little high, but good levels of protein, calcium, and other nutrients redeem these snacks.

Barbara's Organic 100 Calorie Mini Cookies Packs Free of artificial flavors, colors, and preservatives.

WORKING OUT
at work

Do you avoid excercise during the workday because it's too time-consuming? No more excuses! With this program, you won't even have to change your clothes or shower.

MAKE IT A HABIT
Curb All-Day Nibbling

 Grazing may be causing you to pack on the pounds at work, and you may not even realize it. Try to catch yourself before you "taste-test" your coworker's latest cookie creation or dip into the office candy jar. If you're really hungry (and not eating because you're bored, tired, or stressed), choose something calorie-controlled and filling (see page 121 for Drop 5 options). Also try chewing sugarless gum, which provides the satisfaction of chewing without the calories.

25-Minute At-Work Workout

Start by changing into comfortable shoes that provide arch support. Then get up and walk the halls at work at a moderate pace for 15 consecutive minutes a day, and you'll burn about 60 calories. To stretch, build strength, and get some aerobic activity, add the following:

• **STAIR WALKING (FOR FIVE MINUTES)**

• **WINDMILL STRETCH (FOR ONE MINUTE)** Stand with your feet twelve inches apart and your arms stretched straight out to your sides. Then bend at the waist and touch your right hand to your left foot. Return to original position, and touch your left hand to your right foot, then return to original position again. Continue stretching gently—if you can't reach your foot, reach as far as you can without discomfort.

• **WALL PUSH-UPS (FOR TWO MINUTES)** Stand facing a wall with your feet shoulder-width apart and your toes about two feet from the wall. Place your palms flat against the wall with your hands shoulder-width apart and at shoulder height. Keeping your feet stationary and your back straight, count to three as you bend at the elbows, moving your body toward the wall. Count to three again as you push away from the wall. Repeat.

• **CHAIR SQUATS (FOR TWO MINUTES)** Stand with your back to a sturdy stationary chair, your feet about shoulder-width apart, your heels about one foot in front of the chair, and your arms straight out in front of you, parallel to the floor. Lower your body to a seated position, count to three and stand back up to the starting position. Repeat. Try to achieve a 90-degree angle with your legs when you move to the seated position. Once you become stronger, try not to sit at all during the exercise.

Take a Quick Walk

A California State University study that tracked frequent snackers found that those who went for a brisk five-minute walk when they felt frazzled were much less likely to grab a candy bar than those who just sat at their desks. "Walking for only a few minutes lifts serotonin levels—and that boosts your mood and leaves you feeling less anxious," explains Robert Thayer, PhD, professor of psychology at California State University. Keep an extra pair of sneakers at your workplace and start moving! Go for a walk around the block or, if it's difficult to get out, stroll around your office or climb a few flights of stairs.

Learn from the "Losers"

"I use my lunch hour every day to get in 60 minutes of walking."

—LISA SKILES,
100 POUNDS LOST

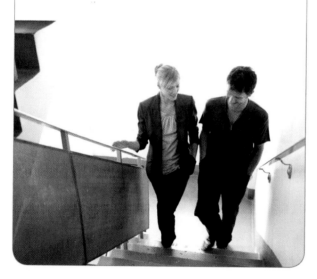

BEFORE

AFTER

STAY
on track

If you want to Drop 5, consistency is your ally. From relying on sticky-note reminders to rewarding yourself for good behavior, here are tips and tricks that will help you stay the course.

DIET TRAP
Skimping on Sleep

Work deadlines, family commitments, and busy schedules—all eat into your time. Multiple studies have shown that sleeping too little increases appetite, compromises insulin sensitivity (which can lead to weight gain), and affects other hormones that control hunger. If you're coming up short on the recommended seven to nine hours a night, turn off the TV/smartphone/computer and get to bed earlier. Plan your life (including your work life) to ensure you get the shut-eye you need each night.

Would You Lose Weight for Money?

Get paid to Drop 5. It sounds like a scam, but a town in Italy is making a deal with its residents to lose weight and gain a few Euros in exchange. Corporations in America have offered such incentives to their employees, knowing that it will cost them less money now than paying for weight-related health problems later. If you were offered money to shed weight, could you do it, and would the incentive make it any easier? If you're intrigued by the idea, talk to the HR director in your workplace to discuss options. Check out the websites Fatbet.net and Makemoneylosingweight.com; both are designed for dieters who want to challenge one another. The site stickK.com facilitates personal commitment contracts for weight loss so you can make a weight-loss wager with some work pals.

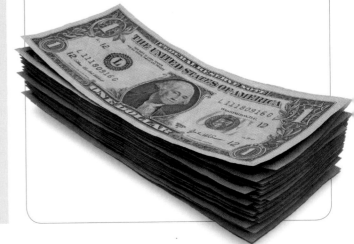

BREAK BAD WORKPLACE PATTERNS

Find your eating type at work, then learn the tricks to eat better.

STYLE	BEHAVIOR	TIPS
Grazer	You can't walk through the teacher's lounge without grabbing a doughnut or Danish, or you regularly pick up treats in the office kitchen. You often snack out of habit, not hunger.	Keep low-cal, nutritious items like grapes, baby carrots, and berries at hand so you can graze without the damage. Eat only in designated areas (in the lunch room, for example)—not in meeting rooms, your cubicle, or in the halls.
Stuffer	You have what grandmas call a healthy appetite. Though you rarely snack in the office, at mealtime you clean your plate and often go for seconds.	Instead of eating until you're stuffed, tune in to your body for cues that tell you you're no longer hungry—it takes practice to become more aware.
Party Binger	You're good at watching your food choices, except at office social events. At coworkers' birthday parties and client events, for example, you pay no attention to how much you're consuming.	Chew sugar-free gum or mints at events to keep your mouth occupied and as a reminder to watch what you eat. When you're chatting with someone, set your food aside. If you don't, you could eat every bite without tasting any of it.

Drop

5 DO IT NOW Use Sticky Notes as Healthy Reminders Sometimes, in the middle of a **busy workday,** you can lose all sense of reality and rationalize your way into eating something super **high calorie** or skipping a workout. To **avoid this,** try posting positive **sticky notes** on your computer, your file cabinets, and your desk that say, "Drink **more water!**" or "Eat an apple, not a cookie" or "Have a piece of chocolate, not a slice of chocolate cake" or "Go for **a walk**—you'll be happy you did!"

DIET TRAP
Discounting the Little Things

It's easy to believe they don't make a difference. But just six 5-minute walks a day burn off about 100 calories, which translates into 10 pounds shed in a year.

- Park your car farther away from your workplace.

- If you take the bus, get off a few stops early and walk the last few blocks.

- Take several 5-minute walking breaks during the day. Walk around the school (teachers), the store (retail workers), the floor (office employees), or the neighborhood (if you work from home).

- Stretch or do light strengthening exercises at your desk.

- Hold walking meetings outdoors (you can talk *and* walk!).

- Take the long route every time you go to the restroom, copy machine, a coworker's office, a classroom, etc.

- Sit on a stability ball at your desk for an hour or two a day.

- Walk around or pace while talking on the phone.

Say "Om"

A demanding work environment with deadlines and pressure to perform can eat away at your motivation and morale—and your weight-loss efforts. Destressing from everyday work issues can be a powerful way to whittle down. A study from the Oregon Health and Science University found that overweight women who performed relaxation techniques such as meditation, yoga, or even writing in a diary for twenty minutes daily lost an average of ten pounds after eighteen months—without consciously dieting. "We suspect that these techniques helped serve as a buffer to stress, so the women were less likely to overeat," explains study author Anne Nebrow, MD.

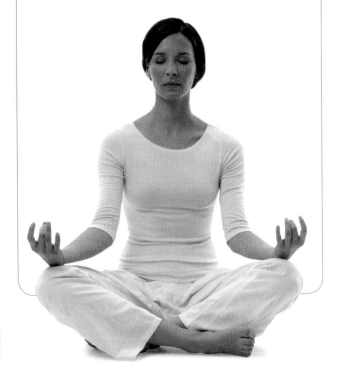

THE DISH ON THE CANDY DISH

Before you dig into the office sweets jar again, check out the calorie savings if you limit your visits to once versus several times a day.

	DIET MADNESS	DIET MAKEOVER	YOU SAVE	SWAP 5 DAYS A WEEK
M&M'S	HIT THE DISH **3 TIMES** 156 CALORIES FOR 54 M&M'S	HIT THE DISH **1 TIME** 52 CALORIES FOR 18 M&M'S	**104** CALORIES	Drop 1 lb in **7** WEEKS
HERSHEY'S MINIATURES CHOCOLATE BARS	HIT THE DISH **3 TIMES** 126 CALORIES FOR 3 MINI BARS	HIT THE DISH **1 TIME** 42 CALORIES FOR 1 MINI BAR	**84** CALORIES	Drop 1 lb in **8½** WEEKS
JELLY BEANS	HIT THE DISH **3 TIMES** 120 CALORIES FOR 30 JELLY BEANS	HIT THE DISH **1 TIME** 40 CALORIES FOR 10 JELLY BEANS	**80** CALORIES	Drop 1 lb in **9** WEEKS
HERSHEY'S KISSES	HIT THE DISH **3 TIMES** 75 CALORIES FOR 3 KISSES	HIT THE DISH **1 TIME** 25 CALORIES FOR 1 KISS	**50** CALORIES	Drop 1 lb in **14** WEEKS
TOOTSIE ROLLS	HIT THE DISH **3 TIMES** 69 CALORIES FOR 3 CANDIES	HIT THE DISH **1 TIME** 23 CALORIES FOR 1 CANDY	**46** CALORIES	Drop 1 lb in **15** WEEKS

In-Box Inspiration

Think of it as your personal trainer (or virtual mom): Every week, you receive a motivational e-mail encouraging you to meet fitness and healthy-eating goals. When 351 office workers tried the Alive! program for four months, their habits improved measurably compared with 436 who didn't get the e-mails. Those who received exercise messages increased their activity by nearly an hour each week, while people who were reminded to eat more produce upped their consumption by more than ½ cup daily.

You can sign up for Alive! at NutritionQuest.com.

MAKE IT A HABIT
Keep Water at Your Desk (and Drink It!)

We all know that H_2O, at zero calories, is the best diet drink. Here's more evidence: When Stanford researchers analyzed the diets of 173 overweight women, they found that those who drank six glasses a day consumed about 200 fewer calories than their water-skimping peers. Why? Opting for water eliminates the waist-widening calories you'd have taken in with other drinks, say experts. To add some flavorful zing to your water, infuse it with citrus slices or a sprig of mint.

Drop

5 **DO IT NOW Reward Yourself** Motivational experts advise **acknowledging good behavior,** not your results. For example, a package of vending-machine cookies might cost you 300 calories and a couple of dollars. If you treat yourself four times a month instead of twenty, you'll save 4,800 calories and $32. Put a Drop 5 **reward jar** on your desk and set up your own personal acknowledgment system. Then, watch the **money pile** up (instead of the pounds!) and use the extra cash on something fun, like a pair of **earrings** or a **pedicure.**

Drop

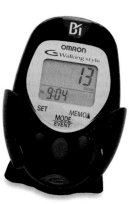

5 DO IT NOW
Pick up Dried Plums (a.k.a. Prunes)

Packed with antioxidants, **potassium,** and fiber, Sunsweet Ones prunes are **surprisingly delicious.** And the individually wrapped dried plums are only **25 calories** each. Snack on four prunes instead of a candy treat, like Snickers (280 calories), and you'll save 180 calories.

Take Frequent Breaks

Standing by the water cooler may help you stay trim. When researchers from the University of Queensland in Australia strapped an accelerometer (a device that measures not just steps but any movements) onto 168 healthy and active men and women for one week, they found that those who incorporated more breaks, like standing or walking around, into their workdays were about 2.3 inches slimmer around the waist than those who parked it in their swivel chairs for hours on end. Breaks were as short as one minute (very doable!) and defined as anything but sitting. So touch your toes at your desk, get up while on the phone, or at the very least, stand up and stretch from time to time.

Learn from the "Losers"

"Exercise, even if it's only for ten minutes. Anything is better than nothing."

—DONNA LENNART, 83 POUNDS LOST

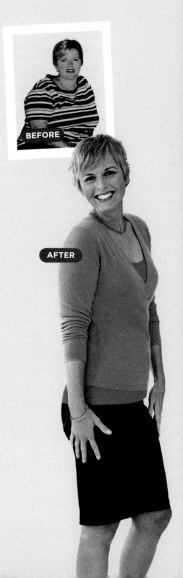

BEFORE

AFTER

WORKING ON
the road

Business travel does not have to derail your Drop 5 efforts. Just put these tips into practice when work travel disrupts your usual routine.

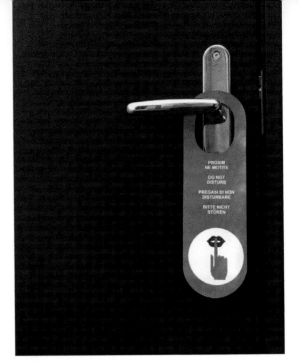

Turn Your Hotel Room into a Gym

If the hotel doesn't have a fitness center, you can turn your room into one. Pack resistance bands and a jump rope, and use filled water bottles as substitutes for light weights. You don't need fancy equipment for push-ups, sit-ups, lunges, or triceps dips (use a chair). If you travel with your laptop or PDA, you can even go online to sites for videos of guided workouts (see page 197 for recommendations). It's like having your own personal trainer in your hotel room!

Drop 5

DO IT NOW Hydrate up High Pressurized planes paired with **salty** snacks are **dehydrating.** When the drink cart rolls around, stick with water or club soda and **steer clear** of **high-calorie sodas** and juices.

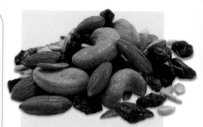

If You've Got a PDA, Make It Work for You

A Stanford University study found that people who used an iPhone or BlackBerry to monitor their fitness routines were more likely to stick to their workouts. The researchers divided 37 nonexercisers into two groups: The first group was prompted twice a day by a personal digital assistant to log their activity level and set exercise goals. Those who didn't respond initially received three more alerts at 30-minute intervals. The second group was given a set of educational handouts on exercise. The alarming difference: The group that got the reminders exercised about five hours per week; the others worked out for only two. For more high-tech help, websites like Traineo.com and NutritionQuest.com deliver motivational diet and exercise tips and goals to your in-box. (See "In-Box Inspiration," page 128.)

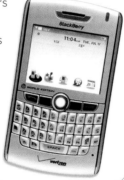

(See "In-Box Inspiration," page 128.)

MAKE IT A HABIT
Pack Snacks

Whether you're hitting the road or taking flight, always try to stash some waist-friendly nibbles in your bag. Fiber-rich bars (see recommendations on page 121), dried fruit, or individually packaged nuts or whole-grain crackers, for example, will help keep your appetite on an even keel. If you're a frequent traveler, keep an extra box of bars or your favorite healthy snack in your suitcase or your car. That way you're always snack-ready, even if you're hurrying the kids out of the house and running to make a flight. Also, search online for healthy places to eat out *before* you travel.

DIET TRAP
Eating When You Are Bored

The tedium of waiting for a delayed flight or a long plane, train, or car ride can drive you to snack. So make sure you keep your brain active—with a book or magazine, crossword puzzle or Sudoku, portable DVD system or MP3 player. You won't even notice you're surrounded by unhealthy foods if you're engrossed in a good movie or novel.

HAPPY HOUR ALERT!

You can enjoy a drink with colleagues without sabotaging your diet, but take care—if you're not mindful of what you swallow, you may guzzle more calories than you'd planned.

Many people consider one cocktail to be a glassful, regardless of how many ounces that glass holds. But dietitians use standard sizes to estimate calorie counts—so a single drink at your favorite bar may

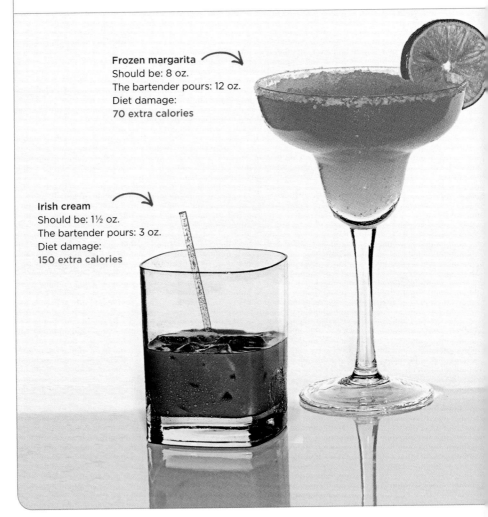

Frozen margarita
Should be: 8 oz.
The bartender pours: 12 oz.
Diet damage:
70 extra calories

Irish cream
Should be: 1½ oz.
The bartender pours: 3 oz.
Diet damage:
150 extra calories

actually be the equivalent of two or three standard-size ones. Before you go out, determine how many calories you're willing to spend on a cocktail and how much that means you can have. If you get a larger pour when you're out with your colleagues, just drink less of it. To familiarize yourself with serving sizes, practice pouring a few drinks using a measuring cup at home. (See also "Drink at Your Own Risk" on page 244.)

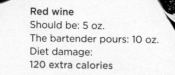

Red wine
Should be: 5 oz.
The bartender pours: 10 oz.
Diet damage:
120 extra calories

Cosmopolitan
Should be: 4 oz.
Bartender pours: 7 oz.
Diet damage:
150 extra calories

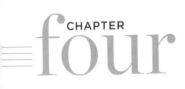

CHAPTER
four

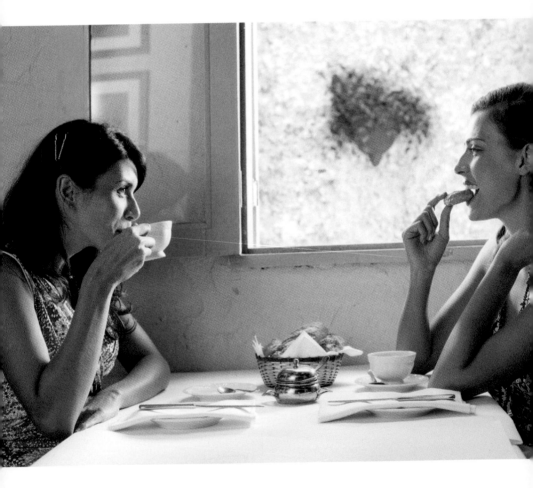

EATING OUT
without blowing
your
diet

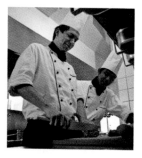

Eating away from home doesn't have to spell trouble for your calorie bottom line. We show you how to keep your waistline in mind, whether you're grabbing fast food or doughnuts or hitting your favorite restaurant.

IT'S NO SECRET THAT DINING OUT can be dangerous for your waistline. When you eat out, your good intentions often fly out the window. After all, it's easy to relax and overindulge when someone else is doing the cooking—and the dishes! Plus, restaurant meals have a lot more calories (at least 60 percent more, according to one recent study) than the same dishes prepared at home. Even professionals can be tricked by hefty portion sizes. When an NYU researcher asked 200 dietitians to estimate the calorie counts of four popular restaurant dishes, the experts low-balled the number for each by a whopping 250 to 700 calories.

While dining out of the house used to be considered a special occasion, in today's fast-paced world in which we're all juggling busy careers, family responsibilities, and social commitments, eating out has become a time- (and sanity-) saving strategy. In fact, the average American eats about five meals outside the home each week, according to the NPD Group, a leading market research firm. The good news: There's always a healthy choice, whether you're at an all-American diner or an ethnic restaurant. Turn the page for the Drop 5 Top 5 things to consider when you're eating away from home.

Drop Top 5

5

EATING OUT HOW-TOS

Frozen Cappuccino
- cinnamon
- amaretto
- vanilla
- hazelnut
- caramel
- gingerbread
- chocolat
- macademia
- naturel

1 GET IN THE KNOW When the California Center for Public Health Advocacy recently asked 523 people to name the healthiest options at popular restaurants, 68 percent didn't get a single answer right. Yikes. Guesstimating nutrition information just doesn't work. Do yourself a favor, and do a little research. Many restaurants post their entire menu plus nutrition information online, making it easy for you to make informed choices ahead of time. If, like most people, you tend to frequent the same spots over and over, go online or ask for in-house nutrition brochures, and find healthy picks at your five favorites. You can also find healthy menu choices for a selection of nearly 30,000 eateries nationwide (from fast food to fancy food) at HealthyDiningFinder.com, which is partly funded by the Centers for Disease Control and Prevention.

And it never hurts to ask your local mom-and-pop eateries for numbers...specifically, calories. It's always a good idea to make healthy out-and-about picks (that is, nutrient-rich meals packed with filling fiber and low in saturated and trans fat, cholesterol, refined sugars, and sodium), but when you are trying to drop pounds, calories are where the rubber meets the road. And keeping your overall calorie intake in mind gives you the freedom to make a less stellar pick (a 250-calorie doughnut, for example) once in a while (see "Test Your Eating Out Calorie IQ" on page 140).

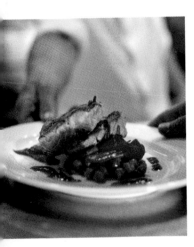

Good news: You can find healthy menu choices for a selection of nearly 30,000 eateries nationwide at HealthyDiningFinder.com.

2 **EAT CONSCIOUSLY** People who manage to lose weight are aware of just how much they eat and drink, and when they overindulge on occasion, they'll make up for it later (see "Practice Damage Control" on page 139). People who struggle with their weight, however, tend to ignore their body's cues and often eat way past fullness. It's easy to get sucked into overeating: Researchers at Cornell University hosted a Super Bowl party for 50 people and served an unlimited number of chicken wings. At half the tables, waiters scooped away the bones as they ate. At the other tables, where partiers could see their scraps piling up, they ate 27 percent less.

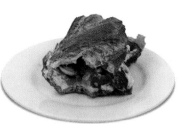

When you are dining out, it's critical to pay attention to your body's cues because portions tend to be extra large. As soon as you start to feel full, stop eating and check your hunger before you have more.

When you are dining out, it's extra important to pay attention to what your body is telling you, since portions tend to be oversized. As soon as you start to feel full, put down your fork, spoon, pastry, or sandwich—stop eating, and give yourself a few minutes to check your hunger before you eat more. Clean plates are not required.

3 **MANAGE YOUR HUNGER** When you skip meals or go hungry in order to save megacalories for a lunch out or social function later in the day, you set yourself up for a dining-out disaster. You'll be so ravenous by the time you get to your dinner, party, or event that you'll end up eating a lot more than if you had had a healthy meal earlier in the day. What's more, skipping meals can result in a slowed metabolism as your "starving" body assumes you are in a state of emergency and starts conserving fat. Keeping yourself satisfied over the course of the day helps to maintain your appetite (and your metabolism) on an even keel, giving you a much better chance to eat consciously, make better choices, and actually enjoy your meals.

4 **FIND BALANCE** You've heard it before, but lots of restaurant foods are full of fat and calories. Some of the worst offenders: cream, cheese, ice cream, butter, baked goods, fried foods, and fatty meats. So how do you make smarter picks? Look for foods that are most like their natural state—fruits, vegetables, beans, and whole grains, rather than chicken nuggets, potato chips, or fruit pies. The better options will contain more vitamins, minerals, antioxidants, phytochemicals, and filling fiber.

But research shows that people who completely ban their favorite foods while trying to lose weight tend to cycle between dieting and bingeing on the foods they restrict. Balancing choices is key. So, if breakfast out at a diner is just not the same without a few strips of bacon,

DAILY CALORIE TARGETS

Consult these guidelines as you choose
recipes, meals, and snacks from this chapter.

FOR WOMEN		FOR MEN	
Breakfast	350	Breakfast	450
Lunch	500	Lunch	600
Dinner	500	Dinner	600
Snack	100	Snack	200
Optional Treat	100	Optional Treat	200
TOTAL	1,450–1,550	Total	1,850–2,050

If you go a little over (or under) at any meal, compensate by adjusting your calories later in the day. Have the optional treat once a day, or save up those calories and have a larger treat every other day, or even two larger 350-calorie treats a couple of days a week. If you want to cut calories a bit more, you can also skip the optional treat altogether.

have them with a cup of oatmeal and fresh fruit. If you can't live without the French fries at your favorite bistro, order grilled fish and veggies as your entrée and share the fries with your dining companion. If you are craving a decadent dessert, share it with a friend (or two or three).

5 **PRACTICE DAMAGE CONTROL** In the real world of dining out and dieting, making the best picks, eating consciously, finding balance, or just saying no (to the bread basket, French fries, dessert, or a second glass of wine) is not always possible. If you occasionally have an indulgent meal—c'mon, it happens—and you still want to Drop 5, you have to be prepared to neutralize the damage. Choose lower-calorie options for your next few meals and increase your activity level for several days, and your indulgence won't have a chance to stick to your hips (or backside or stomach).

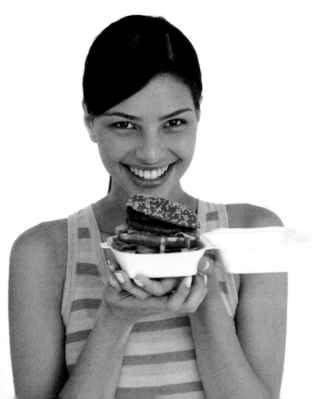

Many restaurants post their entire menu plus nutrition information online, making it easy for you to make informed choices ahead of time.

TEST YOUR EATING OUT
CALORIE IQ
WHICH HAS MORE CALORIES AT...

OUTBACK STEAKHOUSE

Alice Springs Chicken *vs.* **9-ounce Victoria's Filet of Beef?**

The chicken has **1,298 CALORIES**

The beef has **725 CALORIES**

You save 573 CALORIES

RED LOBSTER

Seafood Gumbo *vs.* **Manhattan Clam Chowder?**

The gumbo has **470 CALORIES**

The chowder has **160 CALORIES**

You save 310 CALORIES

PIZZA HUT

3 slices of a 12-inch Fit 'n Delicious Ham, Pineapple, and Diced Red Tomato Pizza *vs.* **6-inch Personal Pan Pepperoni Pizza?**

The ham, pineapple, and tomato pizza slices have **480 CALORIES**

The personal pepperoni pizza has **610 CALORIES**

You save 130 CALORIES

KFC

Mashed Potatoes & Gravy *vs.* **BBQ Baked Beans?**

The mashed potatoes have **120 CALORIES**

The baked beans have **200 CALORIES**

You save 80 CALORIES

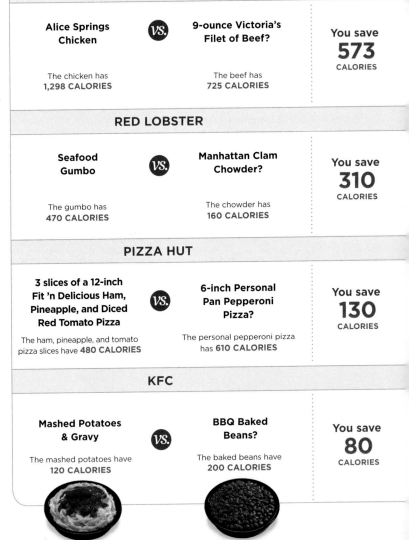

Think you can identify the lower-calorie dishes? See how many you get right. **Bottom line:** It's difficult to spot menu items that are Drop 5 friendly just by their names. Healthy-sounding dishes are often loaded with fat, sugar, and calories.

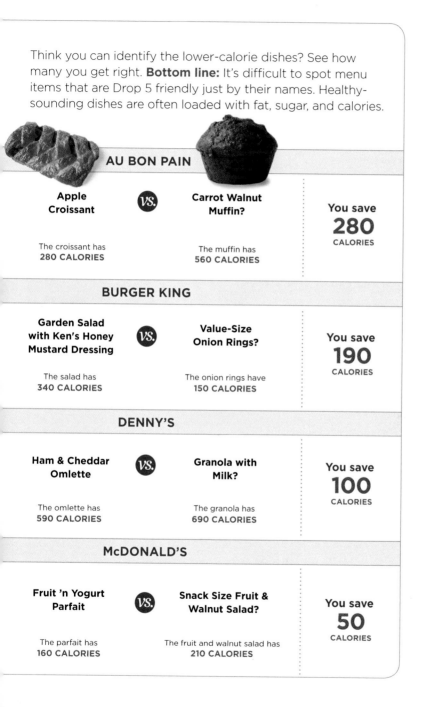

AU BON PAIN

Apple Croissant *vs.* **Carrot Walnut Muffin?**

The croissant has
280 CALORIES

The muffin has
560 CALORIES

You save
280
CALORIES

BURGER KING

Garden Salad with Ken's Honey Mustard Dressing *vs.* **Value-Size Onion Rings?**

The salad has
340 CALORIES

The onion rings have
150 CALORIES

You save
190
CALORIES

DENNY'S

Ham & Cheddar Omlette *vs.* **Granola with Milk?**

The omlette has
590 CALORIES

The granola has
690 CALORIES

You save
100
CALORIES

McDONALD'S

Fruit 'n Yogurt Parfait *vs.* **Snack Size Fruit & Walnut Salad?**

The parfait has
160 CALORIES

The fruit and walnut salad has
210 CALORIES

You save
50
CALORIES

FOOD COURT REPORT

If you're stuck with nothing but the food court, you don't have to derail your diet. Here, the picks that spell trouble—and what to get instead.

BREAKFAST

DIET MADNESS	DIET MAKEOVER	YOU SAVE	SWAP ONCE A WEEK
STARBUCKS Venti White Chocolate Mocha with an Apple Fritter **1,080 CALORIES**	**STARBUCKS** Grande Skinny Vanilla Latte and Perfect Oatmeal with Dried Fruit **370 CALORIES**	**710** CALORIES	Drop 1 lb in **5** WEEKS
DUNKIN' DONUTS Sausage, Egg & Cheese on a Bagel with a Large Mocha Spice Latte **1,090 CALORIES**	**DUNKIN' DONUTS** Egg White Veggie Flatbread with a Small Vanilla Latte Lite **380 CALORIES**	**710** CALORIES	Drop 1 lb in **5** WEEKS
MCDONALD'S Sausage, Egg & Cheese McGriddles with a Hash Brown and a Large Orange Juice **960 CALORIES**	**MCDONALD'S** Fruit 'n Yogurt Parfait with Granola and a Hash Brown **310 CALORIES**	**650** CALORIES	Drop 1 lb in **5½** WEEKS

SNACK

DIET MADNESS	DIET MAKEOVER	YOU SAVE	SWAP ONCE A WEEK
AU BON PAIN Banana Nut Pound Cake **480 CALORIES**	**AU BON PAIN** Small Fruit Cup **70 CALORIES**	**410** CALORIES	Drop 1 lb in **8½** WEEKS
MCDONALD'S Large French Fries **500 CALORIES**	**MCDONALD'S** Vanilla Reduced Fat Ice Cream Cone **150 CALORIES**	**350** CALORIES	Drop 1 lb in **10** WEEKS
TCBY Large Hand-Scooped Chocolate Frozen Yogurt **380 CALORIES**	**TCBY** Small Soft Serve Fat Free Chocolate Frozen Yogurt **80 CALORIES**	**300** CALORIES	Drop 1 lb in **11½** WEEKS
MRS. FIELDS Double Fudge Brownie **360 CALORIES**	**MRS. FIELDS** Chocolate Chip Muffin **80 CALORIES**	**280** CALORIES	Drop 1 lb in **12½** WEEKS

LUNCH | DINNER

DIET MADNESS	DIET MAKEOVER	YOU SAVE	SWAP ONCE A WEEK
PANDA EXPRESS Fried Rice with Beijing Beef 1,420 CALORIES	**PANDA EXPRESS** Mixed Veggies Side, Broccoli Beef, and a Chicken Potsticker 440 CALORIES	**980** CALORIES	Drop 1 lb in **3½** WEEKS
NATHAN'S FAMOUS Chili Dog with Large Onion Rings 1,186 CALORIES	**NATHAN'S FAMOUS** Hot Dog with Corn on the Cob 437 CALORIES	**749** CALORIES	Drop 1 lb in **4½** WEEKS
BURGER KING Whopper with Medium French Fries 1,110 CALORIES	**BURGER KING** BK Veggie Burger with Fresh Apple Fries 425 CALORIES	**685** CALORIES	Drop 1 lb in **5** WEEKS
MCDONALD'S Double Quarter Pounder with Cheese with Medium French Fries 1,120 CALORIES	**MCDONALD'S** Hamburger with a Snack Size Fruit & Walnut Salad 460 CALORIES	**660** CALORIES	Drop 1 lb in **5½** WEEKS
ARBY'S Regular Beef 'n Cheddar Sandwich with Medium Curly Fries 970 CALORIES	**ARBY'S** Regular Roast Beef Sandwich with Applesauce 440 CALORIES	**530** CALORIES	Drop 1 lb in **6½** WEEKS
TACO BELL Grilled Stuft Beef Cheesy Nachos 980 CALORIES	**TACO BELL** Fresco Steak Burrito Supreme and Pintos 'n Cheese 500 CALORIES	**480** CALORIES	Drop 1 lb in **7** WEEKS
WENDY'S Baconator Hamburger with Medium French Fries 1,020 CALORIES	**WENDY'S** Jr. Hamburger with a Small Chili and a Mandarin Orange Cup 540 CALORIES	**480** CALORIES	Drop 1 lb in **7** WEEKS
POPEYES Mild Chicken Breast (with skin), French Fries, and a Biscuit 900 CALORIES	**POPEYES** Mild Chicken Breast (without skin), Mashed Potatoes and Gravy, Corn on the Cob 430 CALORIES	**470** CALORIES	Drop 1 lb in **7½** WEEKS

Drop

5 DO IT NOW Practice Portion Control
Restaurant portions are big. In a recent survey of 300 chefs, many of the cooks copped to serving 12-ounce—or larger—steaks (health professionals recommend 3 ounces) and one to two cups of

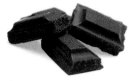

3 ounces fish, poultry, or meat
SIZE OF AN IPHONE
(lean protein is a good choice for dieters, so it's OK to double this serving size to 6 ounces)

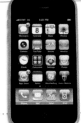

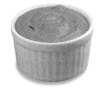

1 ounce cheese or chocolate
SIZE OF ABOUT 4 DICE

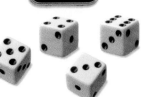

2 tablespoons dressing
THE AMOUNT IN A SHOT GLASS

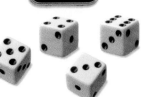

½ cup grains, rice, pasta, or ice cream
SIZE OF A TENNIS BALL

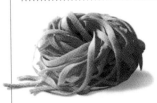

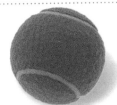

A small dinner roll
SIZE OF A COMPUTER MOUSE

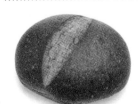

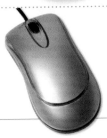

pasta (one serving is half a cup). When you are trying to Drop 5, portion control is key. Use these visual clues to help you avoid portion distortion while dining out. If you are served too much (which is likely), share it or take some home.

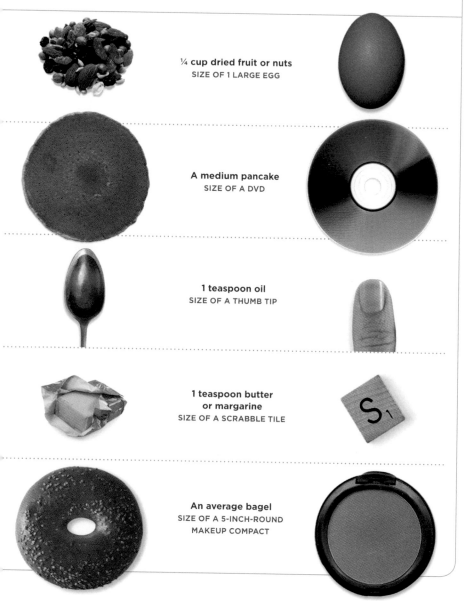

¼ cup dried fruit or nuts
SIZE OF 1 LARGE EGG

A medium pancake
SIZE OF A DVD

1 teaspoon oil
SIZE OF A THUMB TIP

**1 teaspoon butter
or margarine**
SIZE OF A SCRABBLE TILE

An average bagel
SIZE OF A 5-INCH-ROUND
MAKEUP COMPACT

BUILD A BETTER
breakfast

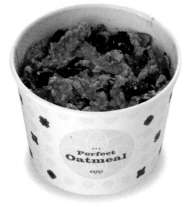

Mornings can be busy, and it's all too easy to simply scarf down the nearest available Danish or doughnut. To help guide you to a healthier breakfast, we list Drop 5 picks from Starbucks and McDonald's and help you navigate other fast-food options. And if you must have your morning doughnut, we supply calorie comparisons so you can make the smartest choice.

STARBUCKS BREAKFAST PICKS

Coffee's not the only jolt at Starbucks. But choose wisely, and you can walk out with a Drop 5 breakfast in hand.

1. **EGG WHITE, SPINACH, AND FETA WRAP** 280 CALORIES

2. **DARK CHERRY YOGURT PARFAIT** 310 CALORIES

3. **PERFECT OATMEAL WITH NUT MEDLEY AND DRIED FRUIT** 340 CALORIES

4. **APPLE BRAN MUFFIN** 350 CALORIES

5. **POWER PROTEIN PLATE** (cheddar cheese, fresh fruit, hard-boiled cage-free egg, mini whole-wheat bagel, and peanut butter) 370 CALORIES

Round out your meal with a low-cal espresso or coffee, either black or with nonfat milk; choose artificial sweetener. Some lattes, cappuccinos, and other specialty coffee drinks are higher in calories and will push you way past your 350-calorie breakfast limit.

DROP 5-FRIENDLY FAST FOOD

Eating on the run does not have to spell disaster for your diet. Here, a cheat sheet to help you avoid major calorie pitfalls—and what to order instead.

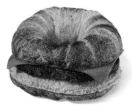

Instead of a Dunkin Donuts Sausage, Egg & Cheese on Croissant...

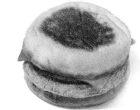

...try an Egg & Cheese on English Muffin

	DIET MADNESS	DIET MAKEOVER	YOU SAVE	SWAP TWO TIMES A WEEK
JACK IN THE BOX	Steak & Egg Burrito 821 CALORIES	Breakfast Jack Sandwich 284 CALORIES	**537** CALORIES	Drop 1 lb in **3½** WEEKS
DUNKIN' DONUTS	Sausage, Egg & Cheese on Croissant 640 CALORIES	Egg & Cheese on English Muffin 320 CALORIES	**320** CALORIES	Drop 1 lb in **5½** WEEKS
McDONALD'S	McSkillet Burrito with Sausage 610 CALORIES	Sausage Burrito 300 CALORIES	**310** CALORIES	Drop 1 lb in **5½** WEEKS
BURGER KING	Sausage, Egg & Cheese Biscuit Sandwich 550 CALORIES	Ham Omelet Sandwich 270 CALORIES	**280** CALORIES	Drop 1 lb in **6** WEEKS

MYTH BUSTER

Fiction Breakfast pastries are out when you're trying to Drop 5. **Fact** Always passing up foods you love will most likely make you crave them even more. The solution? Indulge on occasion, share morning treats with a friend (or eat just half and save the rest for tomorrow), and make calorie-conscious picks that fit within your daily calorie goals.

DIETING ON DOUGHNUTS

OK, they aren't exactly diet fare, but some have twice as many calories as others. Here are many yummy choices for 250 calories or less.

DOUGHNUT	CALORIES
Dunkin' Donuts Sugar Raised	190
Dunkin' Donuts Glazed	220
Dunkin' Donuts Marble or Maple Frosted	230
Dunkin' Donuts Strawberry or Chocolate Frosted	230
Krispy Kreme Original Glazed or Sugar	200
Krispy Kreme Glazed Cinnamon	210
Krispy Kreme Traditional Cake	230
Krispy Kreme Cinnamon Twist or Maple Iced Glazed	240
Krispy Kreme Glazed Cruller	240
Tim Hortons Maple, Chocolate, or Honey Dip	210
Tim Hortons Blueberry or Strawberry Filled	230
Tim Hortons Boston Cream	250

DO THE MATH

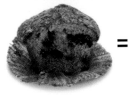

1 Dunkin' Donuts Chocolate Chip Muffin
630 CALORIES

=

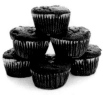

6⅓ Deep Chocolate VitaMuffins
100 CALORIES EACH

Drop 5 Solution

Have a VitaMuffin instead of the Dunkin' Donuts muffin.
100 CALORIES

You Save
530
CALORIES

DOING IT DINER STYLE

Eating at a greasy spoon does not have to wreak havoc on your waistline. Here, what to avoid—and how to customize your order instead.

Instead of a Lumberjack Slam with Syrup... → **...try two Hearty Wheat Pancakes with Sugar-Free Syrup**

	DIET MADNESS	DIET MAKEOVER	YOU SAVE	SWAP ONCE A WEEK
PERKINS	Everything Omelette 1,640 CALORIES	Garden Mix Omelette with a Side of Bacon 365 CALORIES	**1,275** CALORIES	Drop 1 lb in just under **3** WEEKS
PERKINS	Classic Eggs with Bacon 1,420 CALORIES	2 Eggs with Canadian Bacon and Fresh Fruit 330 CALORIES	**1,090** CALORIES	Drop 1 lb in **3** WEEKS
DENNY'S	Heartland Scramble 1,150 CALORIES	2 Scrambled Egg Whites with 4 Slices of Turkey Bacon, a Low-Fat Yogurt, and Seasonal Fruit 356 CALORIES	**794** CALORIES	Drop 1 lb in **4½** WEEKS
DENNY'S	Lumberjack Slam with Syrup 993 CALORIES	2 Hearty Wheat Pancakes with Sugar-Free Syrup 333 CALORIES	**660** CALORIES	Drop 1 lb in just under **5½** WEEKS

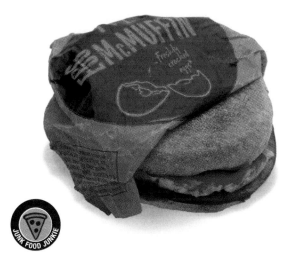

McDONALD'S BREAKFAST PICKS

Yes, it's possible to order a Drop 5 breakfast at McDonald's. Choose from among these calorie-controlled options.

1. **EGG MCMUFFIN AND APPLE DIPPERS** (hold the caramel dip) **330 CALORIES**

2. **FRUIT 'N YOGURT PARFAIT** (without granola), **A HASH BROWN, AND A SMALL NONFAT CAPPUCCINO 340 CALORIES**

3. **2 SCRAMBLED EGGS, A HASH BROWN, AND APPLE DIPPERS** (hold the caramel dip) **350 CALORIES**

4. **FRUIT 'N YOGURT PARFAIT** (with granola) **AND AN ENGLISH MUFFIN WITH A PAT OF WHIPPED MARGARINE 360 CALORIES**

5. **SAUSAGE MCMUFFIN 370 CALORIES**

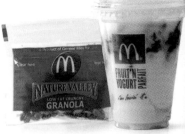

COFFEE DRINK MAKEOVER

If you want to have your latte and Drop 5 too, order the smallest size, skip the sugary syrups (order sugar-free syrup or use artificial sweetener instead) and calorie-laden whipped toppings, and opt for nonfat or low-fat milk.

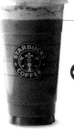

Instead of a Venti Vanilla Frappuccino Blended Coffee with Whipped Cream... ...**try a Tall Vanilla Frappuccino Light Blended Coffee, No Whip**

	DIET MADNESS	DIET MAKEOVER	YOU SAVE	SWAP ONCE A DAY
DUNKIN' DONUTS	Large Coffee Coolatta with Cream **800 CALORIES**	Small Coffee Coolatta with Skim Milk **210 CALORIES**	**590** CALORIES	Drop 1 lb in just under **1** WEEK
STARBUCKS	Venti Vanilla Frappuccino Blended Coffee with Whipped Cream **530 CALORIES**	Tall Vanilla Frappuccino Light Blended Coffee, no Whip **140 CALORIES**	**390** CALORIES	Drop 1 lb in just under **1½** WEEKS
STARBUCKS	Venti Caramel Macchiato with Whole Milk **340 CALORIES**	Tall Skinny Caramel Latte **90 CALORIES**	**250** CALORIES	Drop 1 lb in **2** WEEKS
STARBUCKS	Large Caramel Latte with Whole Milk **330 CALORIES**	Small Latte with Nonfat Milk **90 CALORIES**	**240** CALORIES	Drop 1 lb in just over **2** WEEKS

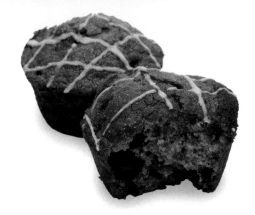

Learn from the "Losers"

"I never deprive myself; I just make great substitutions. For example, I don't go to Dairy Queen (their Blizzards range from 12 to 22 Weight Watchers points, or 520 to 950 calories), but I will get a reduced-fat vanilla ice cream cone at McDonald's (only 3 Weight Watchers points, or 150 calories)."

—MARYKAY BERRY,
150 POUNDS LOST

"When I'm dining out, I always ask the waiter for a 'to go' box before I start eating. That way I can split my portion in half immediately, so I'm not tempted to overindulge. As a bonus, there are tasty leftovers the next day!"

—KAREN EBBESMEYER,
126 POUNDS LOST

BEST IN BAKERY

Pair the following (300-calorie or under) muffins, croissants, or other goodies with a side of fresh fruit, and you'll Drop 5 without feeling deprived.

BAKED GOOD	CALORIES
Au Bon Pain Apple Croissant	280
Au Bon Pain Low-Fat Triple Berry Muffin	300
Corner Bakery Iced Cinnamon Scone	230
Corner Bakery Chocolate Chip Scone	260
Panera Bread Pastry Ring (with apple, cherry, or cheese filling)	220
Panera Bread Chocolate Chip Muffie	280
Starbucks Petite Vanilla Bean Scone	140
Starbucks Blueberry Oat Bar	250

The High Cost of a Coffee Break

People who sip gourmet coffee drinks like lattes and Frappuccinos two or three times a week may take in 260 more calories and 8 teaspoons more sugar per day than those who don't, say researchers from Simmons College in Boston. And it's no wonder. At coffee houses, including the coffee giant Starbucks, doughnut stores, and, now, fast-food chains, low-calorie cups of coffee have morphed into 400-plus calorie monsters. Take a look at the shocking caloric values of some popular drinks.

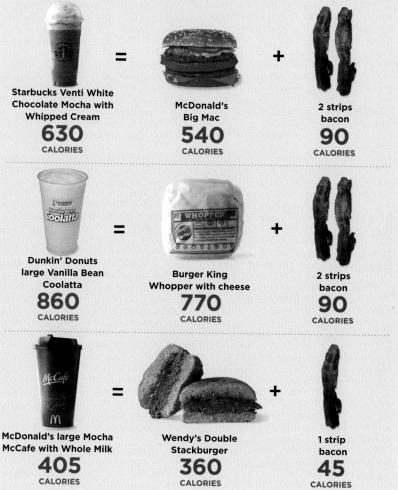

Starbucks Venti White Chocolate Mocha with Whipped Cream
630 CALORIES

=

McDonald's Big Mac
540 CALORIES

+

2 strips bacon
90 CALORIES

Dunkin' Donuts large Vanilla Bean Coolatta
860 CALORIES

=

Burger King Whopper with cheese
770 CALORIES

+

2 strips bacon
90 CALORIES

McDonald's large Mocha McCafe with Whole Milk
405 CALORIES

=

Wendy's Double Stackburger
360 CALORIES

+

1 strip bacon
45 CALORIES

Order à la Carte
Choosing individual items for your morning meal helps you control calories *and* enjoy the foods you crave. Here is how to order "by the menu" at Denny's.

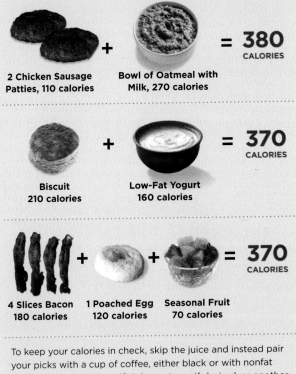

2 Chicken Sausage Patties, 110 calories + **Bowl of Oatmeal with Milk, 270 calories** = **380** CALORIES

Biscuit 210 calories + **Low-Fat Yogurt 160 calories** = **370** CALORIES

4 Slices Bacon 180 calories + **1 Poached Egg 120 calories** + **Seasonal Fruit 70 calories** = **370** CALORIES

To keep your calories in check, skip the juice and instead pair your picks with a cup of coffee, either black or with nonfat milk, sweetened with artificial sweetener if desired, or another noncaloric drink like unsweetened iced or hot tea.

Smoothie Know-How

It can be diet-friendly or a calorie-packed breakfast bomb.

- A Jamba Juice 22-ounce Peanut Butter Moo'd has **770 CALORIES**

- A Smoothie King 40-ounce The Activator Strawberry has **1,112 CALORIES**

- An Orange Julius 32-ounce Tropical Fruit Drink has **690 CALORIES**

Look for smoothies with 400 calories (or fewer) made with some combination of real fruit, fruit juice, low-fat milk, soy milk, yogurt, ice, and no added sugar. Jamba Juice Jamba Light or All Fruit, Smoothie King Trim Down, and Orange Julius Light smoothies are lower-calorie options, but remember, the smaller the size, the better. A 40-ounce Smoothie King Slim-N-Trim Strawberry Smoothie, for example, has 750 calories; choose a 20-ounce to cut your calories in half.

Strawberry Mania

Instead of going out, whip up this pink smoothie, made doubly delicious with its double dose of strawberries.

Total time 5 minutes
Makes 1¾ cups

- ¼ **cup cranberry juice cocktail, chilled**
- 1 **container (8-ounces) low-fat strawberry yogurt**
- 1 **cup frozen strawberries**

In blender, combine cranberry juice, yogurt, and strawberries and blend until mixture is smooth and frothy. Pour into 1 tall glass.

EACH SERVING: ABOUT 326 CALORIES, 10 G PROTEIN, 68 G CARBOHYDRATE, 4 G TOTAL FAT (2 G SATURATED), 15 MG CHOLESTEROL, 141 MG SODIUM, 3 G FIBER

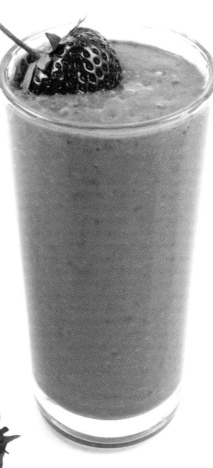

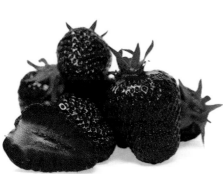

BEYOND THE
brown bag

Packing your own lunch isn't always practical or even possible. Here's how to avoid Drop 5 diet bombs at the deli, salad bar, sub shops, and more.

SANDWICH DO'S

Deli sandwiches are fast and convenient, but you pay the price in fat and calories. Make your stop at the deli counter a Drop 5 Do.

DO...ORDER LEAN FILLINGS. Roast beef, ham, turkey, and chicken breasts have half (or less) the calories and fat of pepperoni, salami, bologna, pastrami, and hard cheeses such as Swiss, cheddar, and provolone.

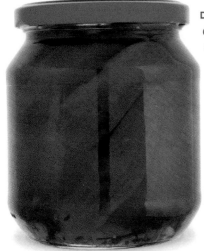

DO...PILE ON VEGETABLES. Fresh (like arugula, spinach, tomatoes, and cucumbers), and roasted (such as onions, peppers, and eggplant), as well as pickles and sauerkraut, are all low-calorie choices.

DO...SKIP THE MAYO, pesto, horseradish sauce, dressings, and "special" sauces and opt for mustard, relish, or salsa instead.

DO...GET YOUR SANDWICH ON FIBER-RICH 100% whole-wheat or whole-grain bread (be sure to ask the sandwich maker). Not only is this a healthier pick, the fiber is filling too.

DO...BE WARY OF CALORIE-LADEN tuna or chicken salads made with mayonnaise; they contain 100 calories per tablespoon.

WINNING LUNCHES

Combining smaller portions of soup, salad, and sandwiches at bakery chains can result in slimming midday meals. These combos add up to around 500 calories.

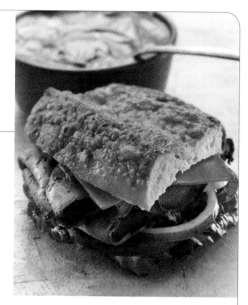

PANERA BREAD

- Half of an Asiago Roast Beef Sandwich (**350 CALORIES**) paired with a cup of Low-Fat Vegetarian Black Bean Soup (**110 CALORIES**)

- Half of a Mediterranean Veggie Sandwich (**300 CALORIES**) paired with half of a Greek Salad (**190 CALORIES**)

AU BON PAIN

- A Demi Ham Sandwich on Baguette (**330 CALORIES**) paired with a small Butternut Squash and Apple Soup (**140 CALORIES**)

- A Demi Tuna Sandwich on Baguette (**330 CALORIES**) paired with a Side Garden Salad with Lite Ranch Dressing (**200 CALORIES**)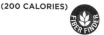

COSÌ

- Half of a Così Market Turkey with Brie Sandwich (**343 CALORIES**) with a cup of Tomato Basil Aurora Soup (**112 CALORIES**)

- Half of a chicken T.B.M. Sandwich (**346 CALORIES**) with a cup of Moroccan Lentil Soup (**99 CALORIES**)

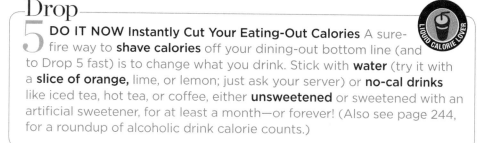

Drop

5 DO IT NOW Instantly Cut Your Eating-Out Calories

A sure-fire way to **shave calories** off your dining-out bottom line (and to Drop 5 fast) is to change what you drink. Stick with **water** (try it with a **slice of orange,** lime, or lemon; just ask your server) or **no-cal drinks** like iced tea, hot tea, or coffee, either **unsweetened** or sweetened with an artificial sweetener, for at least a month—or forever! (Also see page 244, for a roundup of alcoholic drink calorie counts.)

RAISING THE SALAD BAR
High-calorie, fatty salad bar choices abound. Stick to our Top 10 List

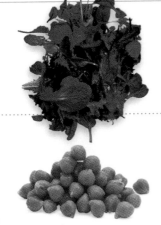

1. LEAFY GREENS
Why? Skip nutrient-poor, boring iceberg, and load up on tastier and healthier lettuces, including spinach, mesclun, and mixed greens.
How much? The sky's the limit.

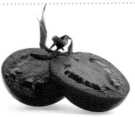

2. BEANS
Why? Loaded with protein, fiber, and nutrients, beans make you feel fuller faster and stay fuller longer. Garbanzo beans and kidney beans are the types most commonly found at salad bars.
How much? Around 2 tablespoons.
40 CALORIES

3. FRESH VEGGIES
Why? Low in calories but high in nutrition and fiber. Go for unprocessed picks (broccoli, tomatoes, green beans, carrots) with lots of color and diversity, and steer clear of calorie-laden dressed vegetable salads such as coleslaw and potato salad.
How much? Keep calorie-dense, starchy veggies (like corn and potatoes) to around ¼ cup
(30 CALORIES); otherwise, there's no limit.

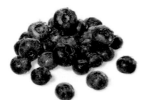

4. FRESH FRUIT
Why? They're low in calories and supply not just tangy flavor, but also phytochemicals, vitamins, minerals, and fiber.
How much? Around ½ cup fresh.
20 TO 60 CALORIES

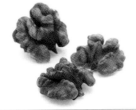

5. NUTS AND SEEDS
Why? Packed with protein and nutrients, they add a wholesome crunch.
How much? Limit to 1 tablespoon to keep calories in check.
45 CALORIES

and you're sure to build a winning weight-loss salad.

6. CHEESE

Why? To increase salad satisfaction, choose a full-fat cheese with more flavor (such as grated Parmesan or crumbled feta or blue cheese), but use it sparingly.
How much? About 1 tablespoon.
25 CALORIES

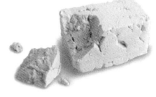

7. OLIVES

Why? Rich in heart-healthy monounsaturated fats and flavor.
How much? A little goes a long way, so limit this calorie-dense pick to around 2 tablespoons sliced or 3 or 4 whole olives.
30 CALORIES

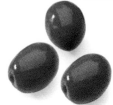

8. HARD-BOILED EGGS

Why? Lots of protein (6 grams per egg), nutrients, and flavor.
How much? Around 2 tablespoons chopped or ½ egg.
30 CALORIES

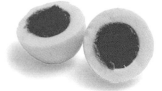

9. GRILLED SKINLESS CHICKEN

Why? A low-calorie, protein-rich choice to help you feel fuller for longer.
How much? Around ¼ cup cubed.
60 CALORIES

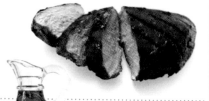

10. LIGHT DRESSING

Why? Full-fat dressings can ruin a perfectly good Drop 5 salad by adding hundreds of unwanted calories; light versions add flavor with minimal calorie impact.
How much? 2 tablespoons.
50 TO 80 CALORIES

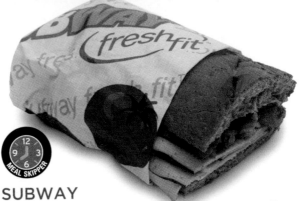

SUBWAY

These calorie counts are based on ordering a 6-inch sub on 9-grain wheat bread.

1. **TURKEY BREAST AND BLACK FOREST HAM** 300 CALORIES

2. **ROAST BEEF** 310 CALORIES

3. **OVEN ROASTED CHICKEN** 320 CALORIES

4. **SUBWAY CLUB** 320 CALORIES

5. **SWEET ONION CHICKEN TERIYAKI** 380 CALORIES

QUIZNOS

Calorie counts here are based on ordering a small.

1. **HONEY BOURBON CHICKEN** 315 CALORIES

2. **TURKEY RANCH AND SWISS** 400 CALORIES

3. **CLASSIC ITALIAN** 505 CALORIES

4. **HONEY BACON CLUB** 460 CALORIES

5. **THE VEGGIE** (guacamole, black olives, lettuce, tomatoes, red onions, mushrooms, mozzarella, cheddar, red wine vinaigrette) **490 CALORIES**

The Sub Story

Sub shops offer a variety of satisfying lunch choices with 500 or fewer calories. The following Drop 5 picks come with dressing and veggies. Consider your 500-calorie lunch budget before you order cheese, chips, drinks, or other extras.

Chicken Done Right

Chicken can be a diet-friendly, fast-food lunch pick, but only if you order the right item. Here's how:

Instead of a KFC Extra Crispy Chicken Breast...

➡️

...try a KFC Grilled Chicken Breast

	DIET MADNESS	DIET MAKEOVER	YOU SAVE	SWAP ONCE A WEEK
WENDY'S	Chicken Club Sandwich **630 CALORIES**	Grilled Chicken Go Wrap **250 CALORIES**	**380** CALORIES	Drop 1 lb in just over **9** WEEKS
JACK IN THE BOX	Homestyle Ranch Chicken Club Sandwich **700 CALORIES**	Chicken Fajita Pita made with Whole Grain **326 CALORIES**	**374** CALORIES	Drop 1 lb in just over **9** WEEKS
McDONALD'S	Premium Crispy Chicken Club Sandwich **630 CALORIES**	Honey Mustard Grilled Chicken Snack Wrap **260 CALORIES**	**370** CALORIES	Drop 1 lb in **9½** WEEKS
KFC	Extra Crispy Chicken Breast **510 CALORIES**	Grilled Chicken Breast **190 CALORIES**	**320** CALORIES	Drop 1 lb in **11** WEEKS
CHICK-FIL-A	Chicken Salad Sandwich **500 CALORIES**	Chargrilled Chicken Sandwich **300 CALORIES**	**200** CALORIES	Drop 1 lb in **17½** WEEKS

Learn from the "Losers"

"I use a mental trick that I learned from a friend in my Weight Watchers group. He avoids overeating at buffets by planning, as he stands on line, exactly what he's going to put on his plate. So now, when I'm a few blocks away from my favorite Chinese restaurant, I start rehearsing my order—steamed broccoli and chicken. Same thing at the corner deli: I review my apple-not-ice-cream plan as I approach. It works every time."

—DIANA ABDEL-RAHMAN,
83 POUNDS LOST

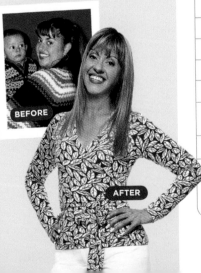

BEFORE

AFTER

SUSHI MIX UP

Mix and match the following Japanese menu items for a healthy Drop 5 lunch.

ROLL (one)	CALORIES
Avocado roll	140
California roll	255
Cucumber roll	135
Eel and Avocado roll	370
Salmon and Avocado roll	305
Shrimp Tempura roll	510
Spicy Tuna roll	290

SUSHI (one piece)	CALORIES
Abalone	45
Bonito	45
Eel	65
Flounder	45
Giant scallop	45
Salmon	50
Shrimp	60
Squid	45
Tuna (bluefin)	50
White tuna (albacore)	55
Whiting	40
Yellowtail	50

OTHER	CALORIES
Edamame (½ cup shelled)	100
Miso soup (1 cup)	40
Soy sauce (1 teaspoon)	10

SLIMMING ON-THE-GO SALADS

Even if you see "garden" in the title, don't assume the dish is low-cal. Here are the fast-food salads to skip, and healthier ones to try instead.

	DIET MADNESS	DIET MAKEOVER	YOU SAVE	SWAP TWICE A WEEK
QUIZNOS	Honey Mustard Chicken Regular Chopped Salad **910 CALORIES**	Pan Asian Regular Chopped Salad **430 CALORIES**	**480** CALORIES	Drop 1 lb in **3½** WEEKS
KFC	Crispy Chicken Caesar Salad with Caesar Dressing and Croutons **650 CALORIES**	Grilled Chicken BLT Salad with Marzetti Light Italian Dressing **230 CALORIES**	**420** CALORIES	Drop 1 lb in **4** WEEKS
BURGER KING	Tendercrisp Chicken Garden Salad with Ken's Honey Mustard Dressing **680 CALORIES**	Tendergrill Chicken Garden Salad with Ken's Light Italian Dressing **330 CALORIES**	**350** CALORIES	Drop 1 lb in **5** WEEKS
AU BON PAIN	Turkey Cobb Salad with Blue Cheese Dressing **640 CALORIES**	Chickpea and Tomato Cucumber Salad with Lite Olive Oil Vinaigrette **340 CALORIES**	**300** CALORIES	Drop 1 lb in **6** WEEKS
WENDY'S	Chicken BLT Salad with Croutons and Honey Dijon Dressing **790 CALORIES**	Chicken Caesar with Caesar Dressing **490 CALORIES**	**300** CALORIES	Drop 1 lb in **6** WEEKS

OUT FOR
dinner

Going out for your evening meal should be a festive occasion, not one that makes you dread the calories you are going to consume. Our Drop 5 tips will help you navigate the menus—from Mexican to Asian to Italian—and make smart picks for appetizers and even dessert!

DIET TRAP
Misbehaving at the Buffet

In a study by Cornell University's Food and Brand lab, twenty-two trained spectators watched 213 diners at eleven all-you-can eat Chinese food buffets in several cities. Patrons who were overweight or obese were more likely than normal-weight patrons to:

- Serve themselves immediately (rather than scan buffet options).
- Choose a large plate.
- Sit facing the buffet.
- Sit without a napkin on their laps.

The take away If you're dining at an all-you-can eat buffet and watching your weight, face away from the buffet, use a small plate, and browse choices before you load your plate. The napkin is up to you!

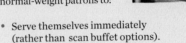

CRAVING 911

Craving	Try This
Chinese fried rice	**Rice with Steamed Veggies**

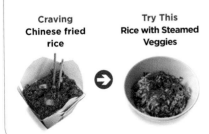

Combine 1 cup cooked white rice, 1 cup steamed vegetables (or a frozen stir-fry variety, cooked), and a splash each soy sauce and Asian sesame oil; toss.

Chinese fried rice
605 CALORIES PER 2 CUPS
Rice with Steamed Veggies
300 CALORIES PER 2 CUPS

You Save
305
CALORIES

RAISING THE STEAKS

The cut of beef you order at a steak house makes the difference between a Drop 5 Do and a dining-out don't. Sirloin steak and filet mignon are by far the leanest picks. They're lower in calories and artery-clogging saturated fat than any other cut (you should have no more than 20 grams of saturated fat per day). Just be sure to pair your lean cut with a side of steamed or roasted veggies like roasted asparagus (around 100 calories), or a side of tomatoes (like a beefsteak tomato salad), instead of typical steak-house sides like steak fries (590 calories) or a baked potato loaded with butter, sour cream, cheese, and bacon (620 calories).

STEAK	BAD (FOR YOUR HEART) FAT	CALORIES	CALORIES PER OUNCE
Sirloin steak (12 OUNCES)	9 g	410	34
Filet mignon (9 OUNCES)	10 g	360	40
Rib-eye steak (12 OUNCES)	16.5 g	563	47
T-Bone steak (16 OUNCES)	28 g	800	50
New York strip (12 OUNCES)	21 g	630	53
Porterhouse steak (20 OUNCES)	40 g	1,100	55
Prime rib (16 OUNCES)	52 g	1,280	80

Drop 5

DO IT NOW Clue into Key Words on the Menu Words like **battered** or **crispy** usually mean the items are fried, while **au gratin, creamed,** and **scalloped** indicate they're loaded with cream or cheese or both (all translate to lots of calories and fat). Terms like **grilled, baked, broiled,** or **roasted** tend to indicate healthier and lower-calorie options.

Attack of the Appetizers

Starters can be diet-stoppers. But chosen with care they can satisfy your cravings and avert a diet debacle. For even greater calorie savings, order one appetizer to share between two people.

Instead of Smoked Mozzarella Fonduta...

...try Mussels di Napoli

	DIET MADNESS	DIET MAKEOVER	YOU SAVE	SWAP ONCE A WEEK
OUTBACK STEAKHOUSE	Aussie Cheese Fries 1,967 CALORIES	Seared Ahi Tuna 431 CALORIES	**1,536** CALORIES	Drop 1 lb in just over **2** WEEKS
CHILI'S	Wings Over Buffalo with Bleu Cheese 1,320 CALORIES	Tostada Chips with Salsa 480 CALORIES	**840** CALORIES	Drop 1 lb **4** WEEKS
OLIVE GARDEN	Smoked Mozzarella Fonduta 940 CALORIES	Mussels di Napoli 180 CALORIES	**760** CALORIES	Drop 1 lb in **4½** WEEKS
ROMANO'S MACARONI GRILL	Shrimp & Artichoke Dip 810 CALORIES	Crab-Stuffed Mushrooms 310 CALORIES	**500** CALORIES	Drop 1 lb in **7** WEEKS

Guiltless Guacamole

We combine creamy mashed white beans with a single avocado for a low-cal dip that's sure to satisfy.

Total time 15 minutes
Makes 3 cups or 12 servings

- 1 **can (15 to 19 ounces) white kidney beans (cannellini), drained and rinsed**
- 1 **tablespoon lime juice, or to taste**
- 1 **jalapeño chile, seeded**
- ½ **cup loosely packed fresh cilantro leaves**
- ¼ **cup coarsely chopped sweet onion (such as Vidalia or Maui)**
- ½ **teaspoon salt**
- 1 **ripe avocado, halved and pitted**
- 2 **plum tomatoes**
  Sliced basil leaves, for garnish (optional)
  Baked tortilla chips or fresh-cut vegetables

1. In food processor with knife blade attached, puree beans and 1 tablespoon lime juice until smooth. Transfer to medium bowl.

2. In same processor, place jalapeño, cilantro, onion, and salt; pulse until juicy and thick.

3. With spoon, scoop avocado from peel into bowl with beans; mash with fork until mixture is blended, with some chunks remaining.

4. Cut each tomato crosswise in half. Squeeze halves to remove seeds and juice. Coarsely chop tomatoes. Stir onion mixture and tomatoes into avocado mixture until blended. If you prefer a little more zip, stir in additional lime juice to taste. Garnish with basil, if you like. Serve with chips or vegetables.

EACH ¼ CUP SERVING: ABOUT 65 CALORIES, 2 G PROTEIN, 8 G CARBOHYDRATE, 3 G TOTAL FAT (0 G SATURATED), 0 MG CHOLESTEROL, 155 MG SODIUM, 3 G FIBER

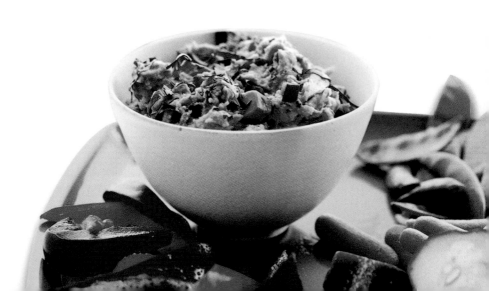

Choose Carefully

Chinese restaurant food is loaded with lots of good-for-your-waist (and heart) picks.

- **Look for...**dishes with vegetables, seafood, tofu, or poultry as the star players. Also, order steamed rice (brown rice if you can find it) instead of fried rice or noodles.

- **Limit...**battered, breaded, or fried anything. Crispy equals fried in Chinese food lingo. Even tofu can turn into a Drop 5 don't after a turn in the deep-fryer. Also, be careful of dishes made with nuts. Although they're healthy, too many nuts makes for too many calories.

- **Share or stash for later...** any leftovers. Chinese food is served family style and designed to serve two or more. Mix your entrée with an order of steamed vegetables to turn it into a lower-calorie and -fat meal. In general, stick with ½ cup of an entrée mixed with 1 cup steamed vegetables served with ½ cup rice.

Wok and Roll!
CHINESE MEAL MAKEOVER

Before you pick up the phone to dial in fried rice and other favorites, check out the calorie counts below—and opt for one of our slimmer Chinese makeovers instead.

MENU MADNESS	MENU MAKEOVER
ORANGE CRISPY BEEF This deep-fried disaster is heavy on the calories but light on the nutrients, as it usually comes sans veggies for a grand total of **1,500 CALORIES**	**BEEF (OR CHICKEN) WITH BROCCOLI** Order beef or chicken with broccoli, and split it with a friend. Serve your half over ½ cup steamed rice, and you'll get a filling, much more waist-friendly meal that contains a good-for-you **550 CALORIES**
COMBINATION FRIED RICE Mix rice with oil, sauce, meat, vegetable, and egg bits, and you get a whopping **1,500 CALORIES**	**STEAMED RICE WITH STIR-FRIED VEGGIES** Order steamed rice and mix a ½-cup serving (100 calories) with half an order of stir-fried mixed vegetables (250 calories), for a healthy, low-cal alternative that's just **350 CALORIES**
GENERAL TSO'S CHICKEN Like other deep-fried Chinese dishes, this battered, breaded, and fried chicken entrée is loaded with fat, calories, and about **1,300 CALORIES**	**MOO GOO GAI PAN** (stir-fried chicken with vegetables) is lower in calories (600) and richer in nutrients than most other Chinese chicken dishes. Eat half an order paired with ½ cup steamed rice for around **400 CALORIES**

Sesame Shrimp and Asparagus Stir-Fry

This Asian-inspired stir-fry is just as tasty as any you'd find dining out, and by making this dish at home you cut the fat by 23 grams and save nearly 700 calories!

Active time 20 minutes
Total time 25 minutes
Makes 4 main-dish servings

- 1 **cup long grain white rice**
- 2 **tablespoons reduced-sodium soy sauce**
- 1 **tablespoon seasoned rice vinegar**
- 1 **tablespoon grated peeled fresh ginger**
- 1 **tablespoon sesame seeds**
- 2 **tablespoons vegetable oil**
- 1 **pound asparagus, trimmed and cut diagonally into 2-inch pieces**
- 1 **pint cherry tomatoes**
- 1 **pound large shrimp, cleaned and cooked**
- 1 **teaspoon Asian sesame oil**

1. Cook rice as label directs.

2. Meanwhile, in cup, stir together soy sauce, rice vinegar, and ginger; set aside.

3. In 12-inch skillet over medium-high heat, toast sesame seeds about 4 minutes or until golden. Transfer to small bowl.

4. In same skillet, heat vegetable oil over medium-high heat until hot. Add asparagus and cook 5 minutes or until tender-crisp, stirring frequently. Add tomatoes and cook 2 minutes, stirring frequently. Stir soy-sauce mixture and shrimp into asparagus mixture; cook 1 minute to heat through. Remove skillet from heat; stir in sesame oil.

5. To serve, spoon rice onto 4 dinner plates; top with shrimp mixture and sprinkle with toasted sesame seeds.

EACH SERVING: ABOUT 370 CALORIES, 31 G PROTEIN, 45 G CARBOHYDRATE, 7 G TOTAL FAT (1 G SATURATED FAT), 221 MG CHOLESTEROL, 455 MG SODIUM, 3 G FIBER

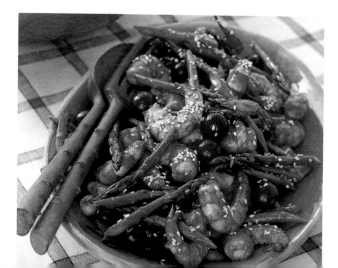

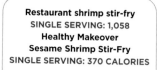

Restaurant shrimp stir-fry
SINGLE SERVING: 1,058
Healthy Makeover
Sesame Shrimp Stir-Fry
SINGLE SERVING: 370 CALORIES

You Save
688
CALORIES

Olé!
MEXICAN MEAL MAKEOVER

How can you make your evening *comida* Drop 5 friendly? Here are some hints.

MENU MADNESS	MENU MAKEOVER
CHICKEN FAJITAS The four fajitas, refried beans, rice, sour cream, and guacamole found on most fajita platters add up to a devastating **1,660 CALORIES**	**FAJITAS MINUS THE SIDES** Skip the typical sides and have just two fajitas paired with an order of beans that aren't fried, and you'll get just **620 CALORIES**
CRISPY CHICKEN TACOS Two deep-fried tacos with refried beans and rice supply **1,040 CALORIES**	**SOFT CHICKEN TACOS** For less fat and fewer calories order two soft tacos (instead of crispy, a.k.a. deep-fried, ones) and skip the sides. **440 CALORIES**
BEEF CHIMICHANGA One of these deep-fried messes paired with refried beans, rice, sour cream, and guacamole adds up to **1,610 CALORIES**	**BEEF ENCHILADA** If it's beef you're craving, order a beef enchilada with a side of Mexican rice, and you'll get just **550 CALORIES**

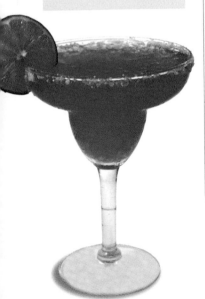

Turkey Fajitas

Fajitas—essentially meat stir-fried and wrapped in warm flour tortillas—are Mexican must-haves. Our version, made with turkey breast meat and without the fatty condiments, knocks more than 1,000 calories off the typical platters found in most restaurants.

Active time: 20 minutes
Total time: 30 minutes
Makes: 4 main-dish servings

- 1 **medium onion (6 to 8 ounces)**
  Olive-oil nonstick cooking spray
- 2 **medium red and/or yellow peppers (4 ounces each), cut into ¼-inch wide slices**
- 1 **pound turkey-breast cutlets**
- ¼ **cup fajita cooking sauce**
- 1 **lime**
- ¼ **cup reduced-fat sour cream**
- 8 **fajita-size flour tortillas (96% fat-free)**

1. Cut onion in half lengthwise, keeping stem intact, then slice from top through stem into ¼-inch strips.

2. Spray grill pan with nonstick cooking spray; heat on medium-high until hot. Spray peppers and onion with cooking spray; place in pan. Cook 12 minutes or until tender and grill marks appear, tossing often.

3. Meanwhile, cut turkey crosswise into ¼-inch-wide strips. In bowl, toss turkey with cooking sauce; set aside.

From lime, grate 1 teaspoon peel. Cut lime into wedges; stir peel into sour cream.

4. Transfer vegetables from grill pan to plate; cover with foil to keep warm.

5. Remove pan from heat; spray with cooking spray. Add turkey and cook on medium-high 6 to 7 minutes or until grill marks appear on the outside and turkey is no longer pink inside (cut into a strip to check), turning once. While turkey cooks, wrap tortillas in damp paper towels; microwave on High 1 minute.

6. To serve, top tortillas with turkey and vegetables; fold over to eat out of hand. Serve with sour cream and lime wedges.

EACH SERVING:
ABOUT 455 CALORIES, 38 G PROTEIN, 65 G CARBOHYDRATE, 6 G TOTAL FAT (1 G SATURATED), 76 MG CHOLESTEROL, 830 MG SODIUM, 9 G FIBER

Restaurant chicken fajitas
SINGLE SERVING: 1,660 CALORIES
Turkey Fajitas
SINGLE SERVING: 455 CALORIES

You Save
1,205
CALORIES

Make It a Drop 5 Meal
Serve with ½ cup nonfat canned refried beans.
COMPLETE MEAL: 555 CALORIES

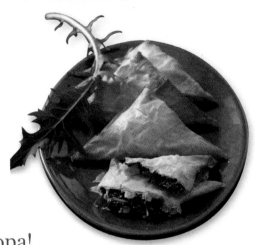

Mediterranean Flavors

Thumbs Up
Dishes like **hummus** (ground garbanzos), **baba ghanouj** (pureed eggplant), **tabbouleh** (a salad of bulgur, tomatoes, and parsley), **souvlaki** (meat or poultry kebabs), **roasted chicken,** and **grilled or broiled fish** offer diners plenty of delicious ways to go Greek while you Drop 5.

Thumbs Down
Gyros (a pita and meat sandwich), **moussaka** (eggplant and meat casserole topped with béchamel sauce), **kefte** (ground meat patties), and **pastitsio** (a sort of Greek meat lasagna) spell big trouble for your waist and heart, delivering close to 1,000 calories and more than a day's worth of artery-clogging saturated fat.

Oopa!
GREEK MEAL MAKEOVER
You can sink your teeth into a Greek meat sandwich and even a savory stuffed pastry. Here's how to do it the Drop 5 way.

MENU MADNESS	MENU MAKEOVER
GYRO SANDWICH This pita bread sandwich stuffed with meat, yogurt sauce, feta, lettuce, and tomato has **760 CALORIES**	**LAMB OR PORK SOUVLAKI SANDWICH** It's made with leaner meat. Pair it with rice for a Drop 5 dinner of **500 CALORIES**
MOUSSAKA An order of this casserole dish along with the typical side of rice will leave you with **1,070 CALORIES**	**SPANIKOPITA** Opt for the spanikopita (pastry stuffed with spinach and cheese) instead. You'll even have room for a few bites of baklava **400 CALORIES**

Greek Chicken Burgers

This delicious burger, made with tangy feta cheese, fresh mint, and ground chicken, is a calorie-saving alternative to a gyro sandwich.

Active Time 20 minutes
Total Time 30 minutes
Makes 4 servings

- 4 (6-inch) pita pockets
- 1 pound ground chicken
- ½ cup crumbled feta cheese
- 1 large egg
- ¾ cup loosely packed fresh mint leaves, chopped
- ¼ teaspoon salt
- ¼ teaspoon ground black pepper
- 6 ounces low-fat plain yogurt
- 4 cups romaine or iceberg lettuce, thinly sliced
- 3 plum tomatoes, sliced

1. Cut off a third of each pita and set pita pockets aside. Grate small pieces on fine side of grater or pulse in food processor to make ½ cup bread crumbs.

2. In large bowl, mix crumbs, chicken, feta, egg, ¼ cup mint, salt, and pepper until just combined. Shape mixture into 8 small ¾-inch-thick burgers.

3. Heat nonstick 12-inch skillet over medium heat. Add burgers and cook 10 to 12 minutes or until browned on both sides and cooked through.

4. Meanwhile, in small bowl, combine yogurt and remaining ½ cup mint. To serve, fill each pita with lettuce, tomatoes, 2 burgers, and yogurt sauce.

EACH SERVING: ABOUT 430 CALORIES, 33 G PROTEIN, 38 G CARBOHYDRATE, 16 G TOTAL FAT (4 G SATURATED), 73 MG CHOLESTEROL, 750 MG SODIUM, 4 G FIBER

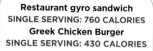

Restaurant gyro sandwich
SINGLE SERVING: 760 CALORIES
Greek Chicken Burger
SINGLE SERVING: 430 CALORIES

You Save
330
CALORIES

Make It a Drop 5 Meal
Serve with ½ cup frozen sweet potato fries, baked
COMPLETE MEAL: 500 CALORIES

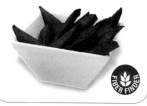

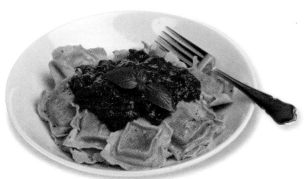

HALL OF SHAME
Pasta Dishes

Diners beware—some of these Italian-style noodles have almost as many calories as you should consume in an entire day.

- Red Lobster Crab Linguine Alfredo
  1,120 CALORIES

- Romano's Macaroni Grill Pollo Limone Rustica
  1,200 CALORIES

- Olive Garden Spaghetti & Italian Sausage
  1,270 CALORIES

- Outback Steakhouse No Rules Parmesan Pasta
  1,379 CALORIES

- Ruby Tuesday Chicken & Broccoli Pasta
  1,628 CALORIES

Bellissimo!
ITALIAN MEAL MAKEOVER

A bowlful of pasta can serve up a heap of calories. See our makeovers for Drop 5–friendly options to twirl around your fork.

MENU MADNESS	MENU MAKEOVER
FETTUCINE ALFREDO This creamy pasta dish is packed with **1,500 CALORIES**	**LINGUINE WITH WHITE CLAM SAUCE** Ask for a half order plus a side of steamed or roasted veggies. You'll even have room to share a dessert or have a glass of wine because the total is **455 CALORIES**
LASAGNA One order of this layered-meat-cheese-and-noodle Italian classic has **960 CALORIES**	**CHEESE RAVIOLI** with tomato or marinara sauce is a decent, though not very low-cal, choice at **620 CALORIES**

Creamy Mushroom Cavatappi

If you're craving creamy pasta, whip up this quick and easy dish instead of heading out for fettuccine alfredo, and you'll save a whopping 1,100 calories and 89 grams of fat.

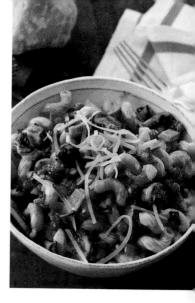

Active time 15 minutes
Total time 30 minutes
Makes 6 main-dish servings

- **12 ounces cavatappi (half moon–shaped pasta; penne can be substituted)**
- **2 teaspoons olive oil**
- **1 small onion (4 to 6 ounces), chopped**
- **1 package (8-ounces) sliced cremini mushrooms**
- **1 tablespoon cornstarch**
- **1½ cups low-fat (1%) milk**
- **½ cup grated Parmesan cheese, plus additional for serving**
- **¼ teaspoon salt**
- **¼ teaspoon ground black pepper**
- **1 (10-ounce) package frozen peas**
- **8 ounces deli-sliced ham, cut into ½-inch-wide strips**

1. Heat large covered saucepot of *salted water* to boiling on high. Add pasta and cook as label directs.

2. Meanwhile, in 12-inch skillet, heat oil on medium until hot. Add onion and cook 3 minutes or until beginning to soften. Increase heat to medium-high, and stir in mushrooms; cook 8 to 10 minutes or until mushrooms are golden and most liquid has evaporated, stirring frequently. Transfer mushroom mixture to small bowl.

3. In 2-cup liquid measuring cup, whisk cornstarch into milk; add to same skillet and heat to boiling on medium, whisking frequently. Boil 1 minute, stirring constantly to prevent scorching. Remove skillet from heat and whisk in Parmesan, salt, and pepper.

4. Place peas in colander. Pour pasta over peas; drain and return to saucepot. Stir in mushroom mixture, cheese sauce, and ham; toss to coat. Serve with freshly grated Parmesan.

EACH 1½-CUP SERVING: ABOUT 400 CALORIES, 23 G PROTEIN, 57 G CARBOHYDRATE, 8 G TOTAL FAT (3 G SATURATED), 28 MG CHOLESTEROL, 880 MG SODIUM, 5 G FIBER

Restaurant fettucine alfredo
SINGLE SERVING: 1,500 CALORIES
Creamy Mushroom Cavatappi
SINGLE SERVING: 400 CALORIES

You Save
1,100
CALORIES

Make It a Drop 5 Meal

Serve with 2 cups mixed greens tossed with 100 calories of dressing.
COMPLETE MEAL: 520 CALORIES

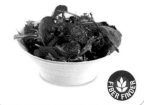

Chain Reaction

Lots of family-style chain restaurants now offer menu options that help you enjoy dinner out without blowing your diet.

- **Applebee's** Under 550 Calories Menu: Good choices include Asiago Peppercorn Steak **(390 CALORIES)** and Spicy Shrimp Diavolo **(500 CALORIES)**

- **Olive Garden** Garden Fare Menu: Good choices include Venetian Apricot Chicken **(380 CALORIES)** and Linguini alla Marinara **(430 CALORIES)**

- **Red Lobster** Lighthouse Menu: Good choices include Wood Grilled Salmon or Rainbow Trout with Broccoli **(265 CALORIES)**

ITALIAN PICKS AND PANS

Delicious and nutritious, our picks help you enjoy the taste without the guilt.

PASTA

Pick	Pan
Pasta paired with red sauces (like marinara and other tomato sauces), clam sauce, vegetables (like pasta primavera made with olive oil, not cream), and grilled chicken or seafood	Pasta paired with cream, cheese, or butter sauces (like Alfredo and carbonara), meat (like meatballs or sausage), and sauces made with meat (like Bolognese)

PIZZA

Pick	Pan
Thin-crust pies with lots of veggies, less cheese (or, even better, no cheese), lean meat (like ham or chicken), and, when available, a healthier whole-grain crust	Deep-dish pies with extra cheese and fatty meat toppings (like sausage, ground beef, pork, or pepperoni) or stuffed crusts

SALADS

Pick	Pan
Mixed green salads loaded with fresh veggies with dressings and cheese on the side (and used sparingly)	Caesar salads, Caprese (mozzarella and tomato) salads, and meat-and-cheese antipasto salads

CLASSICS

Pick	Pan
Simply prepared (broiled and grilled) fish and chicken dishes	Parmigiana dishes (like eggplant, chicken, and veal Parmigiana), dishes loaded with cheese and meat (like manicotti and lasagna), and fried foods (like calamari fritti or mozzarella fritta)

Whole-Wheat Penne Genovese

An onion-flecked white bean sauté adds heft to this fresh and healthy pesto pasta dish, making it light yet satisfying.

Total time 30 minutes
Makes 6 main-dish servings

- **12 ounces whole-wheat penne or rotini**
- **1½ cups packed fresh basil leaves**
- **1 clove garlic**
- **3 tablespoons water**
- **3 tablespoons olive oil**
- **¼ teaspoon salt**
- **¼ teaspoon freshly ground black pepper**
- **½ cup freshly grated Pecorino-Romano cheese**
- **1 small onion (4 to 6 ounces), chopped**
- **1 can (15 to 19 ounces) white kidney beans (cannellini), rinsed and drained**
- **1 pint grape tomatoes (red, yellow, and orange mix if available), each cut into quarters**

1. Heat large covered saucepot of *salted water* to boiling over high heat. Add pasta and cook as label directs.

2. Meanwhile, make pesto: In food processor with knife blade attached, blend basil, garlic, water, 2 tablespoons oil, salt, and pepper until pureed, stopping processor occasionally and scraping bowl with rubber spatula. Add Romano; pulse to combine. Set aside.

3. In 12-inch skillet, heat remaining 1 tablespoon oil on medium until very hot; add onion and cook 5 to 7 minutes or until beginning to soften. Stir in white beans, and cook 5 minutes longer, stirring occasionally.

4. Reserve *¼ cup pasta cooking water*. Drain pasta and return to saucepot; stir in white-bean mixture, pesto, cut-up tomatoes, and reserved cooking water. Toss to coat.

EACH 1⅓-CUP SERVING: ABOUT 375 CALORIES, 15 G PROTEIN, 59 G CARBOHYDRATE, 10 G TOTAL FAT (2 G SATURATED), 5 MG CHOLESTEROL, 435 MG SODIUM, 9 G FIBER

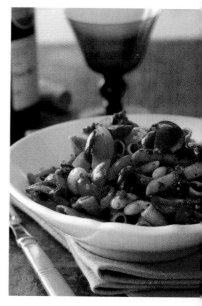

Eat a Treat at Home

Save calories and money: Hold off on dessert until you get back to the house.

ABOUT 120 CALORIES EACH PER SERVING

- 1 cup Italian ice
- ½ cup sorbet
- 6 meringue cookies (make it 5 if you're having chocolate)
- 2 cups berries with 3 tablespoons light whipped dessert topping
- ½ cup Edy's Slow Churned Rich & Creamy light chocolate ice cream

OH-SO-SWEET MAKEOVERS

Don't dash your Drop 5 efforts by ingesting a diet bomb for dessert. Instead, if you must indulge, satisfy your sweet tooth with one of these yummy makeovers—and share it with a friend (or three!) to get your sugar fix for a fraction of the calories and fat.

	MADNESS	MAKEOVER
ROMANO'S MACARONI GRILL	**TIRAMISU** Ladyfingers soaked in espresso, then layered between rich mascarpone cream are a dieter's nightmare at **1,120 CALORIES AND 48 GRAMS OF FAT**	**VANILLA GELATO** Authentic Italian gelato with fresh strawberries is a sensible—and delicious—alternative at **110 CALORIES AND 3.5 GRAMS OF FAT**
CHILI'S	**BROWNIE SUNDAE** Who doesn't love a warm chocolate brownie topped with vanilla ice cream and hot fudge, but this one's a diet sink hole at **1,320 CALORIES AND 68 GRAMS OF FAT**	**SWEET SHOT KEY LIME PIE** A better choice is this little layered dessert served in a shot glass for a sweeter-on-your-waistline total of **240 CALORIES AND 12 GRAMS OF FAT**
RUBY TUESDAY	**ITALIAN CREAM CAKE** Each slice of this buttermilk and walnut cake layered with cream cheese contains a diet derailing **990 CALORIES AND 56 GRAMS OF FAT**	**BERRY GOOD YOGURT PARFAIT** Opt for creamy and crispy layers of yogurt and granola with a blackberry topping for just **162 CALORIES AND 3 GRAMS OF FAT**
RED LOBSTER	**CHOCOLATE WAVE** This rich slice of chocolate cake topped with vanilla ice cream and chocolate sauce will drown your diet in **1,490 CALORIES AND 81 GRAMS OF FAT**	**SURF'S UP SUNDAE** Instead ride a more sensible tide with this classic ice cream sundae, which delivers a more modest **170 CALORIES AND 9 GRAMS OF FAT**

Poached Pears with Fresh Ginger

This do-ahead dessert—with only five ingredients—is fat-free. You'll love the sweet and slightly spicy taste of the poaching liquid.

Active time 20 minutes
Total time 1 hour plus chilling
Makes 8 servings

- 8 **firm but ripe Bartlett or Bosc pears (about 3½ pounds)**
- 1 **cup sugar**
- 1 **(3-inch) stick cinnamon**
- 2 **strips (about 3" by 1" each) orange peel**
- 1 **(2-inch) piece fresh ginger, peeled and cut crosswise into 16 thin slices**
- 6 **cups water**

1. Peel pears. With melon baller or small knife, remove core and blossom end (bottom) of each pear.

2. Place all ingredients in 6- or 8-quart Dutch oven; heat to boiling over high heat. Reduce heat to low; cover and simmer 10 to 20 minutes, until pears are tender. With slotted spoon, transfer pears to large bowl.

3. Heat pear poaching liquid to boiling over high heat; cook, uncovered, over high heat about 15 minutes or until syrup is reduced to about 3 cups.

4. Gently pour hot syrup through strainer over pears. Transfer cinnamon stick, orange-peel strips, and 3 slices ginger to syrup around pears. Cover and refrigerate at least 4 hours or until well chilled, turning pears occasionally. Serve pears with syrup.

EACH SERVING: ABOUT 175 CALORIES, 1 G PROTEIN, 45 G CARBOHYDRATE, 1 G TOTAL FAT (0 G SATURATED), 0 MG CHOLESTEROL, 1 MG SODIUM, 2 G FIBER

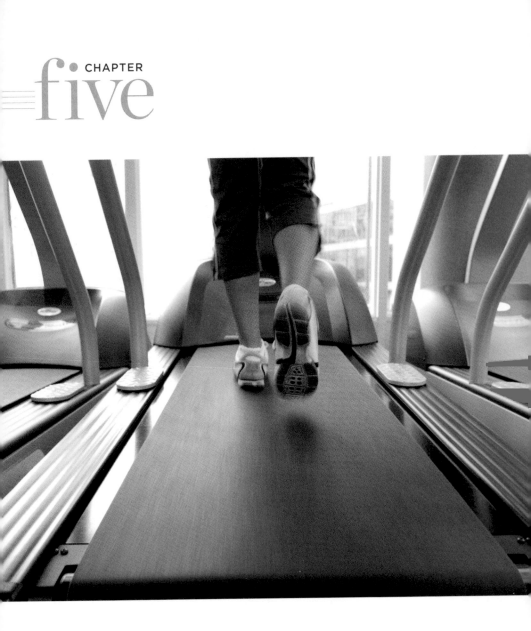

CHAPTER

five

FITNESS FIRST
weight-loss
workout
know-how

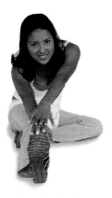

Regular physical activity prevents disease, boosts your mood, relieves stress, and helps you Drop 5 faster.

IF YOU'RE CONFUSED ABOUT HOW MUCH exercise you need to do in order to lose weight, you're not alone. Is it 20 minutes a day—or 30? Or 45? Does it have to be done all at once, or can it be broken up? Should it be aerobic or strength training, and do you need to do a high-intensity workout every time?

While the American College of Sports Medicine and the American Heart Association recommend 60 to 90 minutes of exercise per day for weight management, the truth is, when you are trying to Drop 5, doing any exercise, for any length of time, at any intensity, will help you lose weight faster. Why? Because the more active you are, the more calories you burn. Losing weight boils down to a very simple equation: calories in versus calories out. It's not about gimmicks, fads, or tricks, just basic arithmetic. If you burn more calories than you eat, you will lose weight. So follow the Drop 5 eating advice, add exercise, and you'll see results faster. (Remember, a deficit of 3,500 calories—either because you eat fewer calories or because you burn more calories by working out, or both—will result in a one-pound weight loss.)

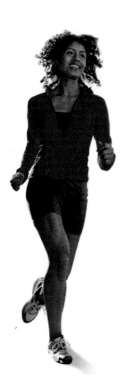

What's more, you'll not only burn calories while you're actively working out, you'll also keep burning them after you've stopped. The secret is muscle building. When you strengthen your muscles, you're creating a calorie-burning machine. Muscle is metabolically active tissue, which means that the more you have, the more calories you burn, even while you're eating dinner with your family, doing the laundry, or relaxing on the couch. In fact, some studies estimate that you burn an additional 35 to 40 calories per day with each pound of muscle you add to your body.

Aerobic exercise, like running, biking, and walking (see page 186 for the "Drop 5 Fat-Blasting Walking Plan") will burn calories and build muscle, as will everyday activities like vacuuming, cleaning house, gardening, and yard work. And if you include strength training (check out the "Drop 5 Twenty-Minute Muscle-Building Plan" on page 192), you will develop even more muscle and work off even more calories.

Here is our favorite Drop 5 workout advice to help you lose weight faster.

MYTH BUSTER

Fiction Your genes determine your metabolism and body weight. **Fact** Only 25 percent of your body weight is determined by your genes—the rest is the result of your behavior. At any time in life, you can drastically change your body weight by combining low-calorie eating and exercise. And you can increase your metabolism at any age by performing strength and resistance exercises.

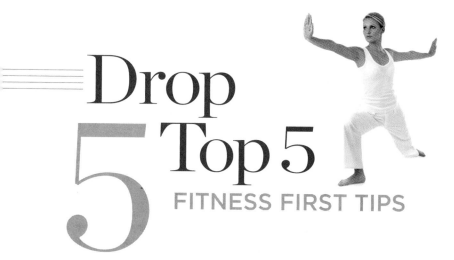

Drop
5 Top 5
FITNESS FIRST TIPS

1 FOLLOW THE PLEASURE PRINCIPLE What do roller skating, hula-hooping, Zumba (Latin rhythm aerobic dancing), kickboxing, and swimming have in common? They're all fun—and they all burn calories while you're doing them. Research shows that when you're enjoying yourself, you're more likely to stick with an activity. And the more you stick with it, the more pounds you'll drop.

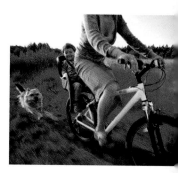

2 EXERCISE FAMILY STYLE "Pick things you can do as a family, like bicycling, hiking, rock climbing, canoeing, or bowling, to keep everyone striving for better health," says Kelli Calabrese, MS, exercise physiologist and fitness consultant. Some local parks may offer fitness courses you could tackle together. Choose a weekend to head to a state park and go hiking. Or check out a local farm and go apple picking. "Take a martial arts class. Everyone's a beginner together; you all start out as a white belt and progress from there," says Calabrese. Or, more simply, toss around a football, go ice-skating, or take a long walk with the dog once or twice a week.

Research shows that when it comes to exercise, if you're doing an activity you enjoy, you're more likely to stick with it. For fun exercise options, complete with calorie counts, see our "Burn, Baby, Burn" ideas sprinkled throughout the chapter.

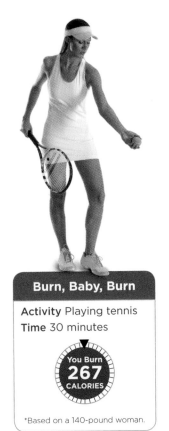

Even if you are not the outdoorsy type, exercise can still be fun for the whole family. With Nintendo's Wii Fit game, even the most committed couch potatoes will enjoy standing on the Wii Balance Board and following on-screen instructions for yoga, aerobics, strength training—even walking a tightrope and hula hooping. You earn points for good performance and get feedback on how you can improve.

3 LEARN A NEW SKILL Always wanted to try in-line skating, golf, cross-country skiing, or ball-room dancing? Would you like to join a softball league or soccer team or take up yoga, tennis, or salsa dancing? Do it! You'll learn something new and Drop 5 at the same time. Check local community organizations or the YMCA for affordable classes. For even more fun, get a group of friends to learn a new, calorie-burning activity together.

4 BREAK IT UP If you don't have a full hour (or even a half-hour) to dedicate to exercise each day, try divvying it up into several mini workouts throughout the day. "Dividing your typical workout in half (say, fifteen minutes in the a.m. and another fifteen at night), or even in thirds (ten minutes a session) isn't just a great way to keep your brain from getting bored: It can give you an even bigger calorie-burning boost," says fitness expert Myatt Murphy, author of *The Body You Want in the Time You Have*. "That's because you'll still burn about the same number of calories while exercising, but after each mini workout, your metabolism stays elevated for roughly 30 to 60 minutes, burning more calories than usual. Do two to three intense, smaller workouts, and your body can burn more calories than it would from a single daily routine."

Burn, Baby, Burn

Activity Playing tennis

Time 30 minutes

You Burn 267 CALORIES

*Based on a 140-pound woman.

Dividing up your workout can even help you stay more dedicated to losing weight. Researchers at the University of Pittsburgh found that people who exercised for ten minutes several times a day were able to exercise an average of 35 minutes longer per week than subjects who were told to do the same amount of exercise in just one session each day. (Consider that the average person who exercises does only the recommended minimum of 20 to 30 minutes, three times a week—about 60 to 90 minutes per week. An additional 35 minutes on top of that is an increase of roughly 33 to 50 percent!) They also burned more calories and improved their cardio-respiratory health.

5 GO AT A REASONABLE PACE Suppose you haven't exercised in a while. After a sudden urge to get fit and lose weight, should you immediately go for a 60-minute run or lift fifteen-pound dumbbells at the gym? Of course not! Doing this will only risk injury. Even if you avoid hurting yourself, you'll be convinced exercise is too difficult and quit before you've really started. The solution? Start slowly and work at an intensity that feels comfortable. Begin with a fifteen-minute leisurely walk, and, when you feel ready, try the "Drop 5 Fat-Blasting Walking Plan" (page 186). Then, branch out and try new activities, whether water aerobics or Tai Chi, nature hikes or bike riding. The best part: The entire time your body is adapting to increased exercise, you're burning calories and on your way to dropping the weight.

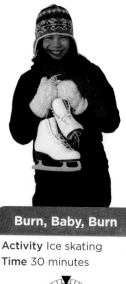

Burn, Baby, Burn

Activity Ice skating
Time 30 minutes

You Burn
184
CALORIES

*Based on a 140-pound woman.

WALK OFF
the weight

You already have the best fat-burning equipment: your feet. The secret is knowing how to use them. Our Drop 5 fat-blasting program will help you find the right pace for *you*— whether that's an easy stroll or a heart-pumping workout. And counting those steps with a pedometer will help ensure that you melt off the pounds.

The Drop
5 FAT-BLASTING WALKING PLAN

Going for a walk may be as easy as putting on your sneakers and stepping outside, but if you want to Drop 5 fast, it's best to have a plan. Our program is specifically designed to bump your body into a higher calorie- and fat-burning zone, so you'll lose weight *and* firm up. Combine this walking plan with the calorie cutbacks, and you could Drop 5 in about 2½ weeks!

You'll do four 30-minute walking workouts a week—ideally on Tuesday, Thursday, Saturday, and Sunday. The step-by-step details are charted out for you on page 188, but here's a quick breakdown of your activities for each day—and how they'll make the weight-loss difference.

TUESDAYS
Walk normally...then speed up for one to two minutes. Go as fast as your feet will carry you, but try to maintain good form (see "Make It a Habit," opposite). This extra "fast lane" push makes your metabolism work overtime so you burn more calories post-exercise.

THURSDAYS
March up inclines If there are hills nearby, choose those that are about a block long. On treadmills, simply increase the incline to about 4 percent. No hills, no treadmill? Get the same muscle boost by walking up one or more flights of stairs for 60 seconds.

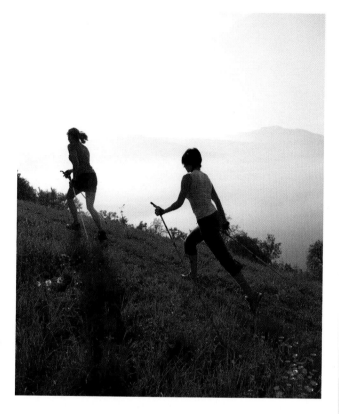

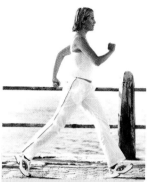

You'll see results fast: Tufts University researchers reported that older adults who added lean muscle tissue through resistance exercises three days a week for twelve weeks boosted their resting metabolism by about 7 percent.

SATURDAYS

Take a brisk walk to build stamina and strength. Find a pace that's quick enough for you to feel a burn, but not so tough that you can't sustain it for at least twenty minutes.

SUNDAYS

This is your day of rest. Translation: You can walk as slowly or as fast as you like. Just make sure you get outdoors and hit the pavement.

MAKE IT A HABIT
To Lose More, Walk Right

For a workout that's more than just leg exercise, copy this woman's total-body style:

- Keep your chin up and face forward—don't look down.

- Hold your arms at a 90-degree angle and pump them forward and back, with your hands in loose fists. Stand upright, with your shoulders back and relaxed.

- Always place your heel down first and let the middle of your foot and toes follow.

Find Your Pace

The workout, right, is divided into four pace levels: Easy, Moderate, Challenging, and Hard. But what's easy for one person can be hard for another—you may feel pooped after a brisk walk, while it could take a near jog to get a friend going. How to figure out your best-results speed? Talk as you're walking, and gauge how hard it is for you to speak. Then see where you score on the guide below.

Easy The pace of your walk is so effortless, you can gab freely (no panting, no breathlessness).

Moderate You can still chat, but you need to pause occasionally to catch your breath.

Challenging You have little breath for small talk, but you can still manage to talk in short sentences.

Hard You can get out a *yes, no,* or *maybe.* But you really can't talk right now!

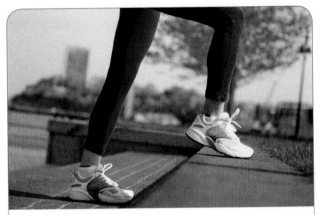

WALKING PLAN CHART

Four 30-minute walks a week will help you Drop 5. Follow this four-week program.

WEEK 1

TUESDAY

- Warm up for 5 minutes at EASY level.
- Increase to HARD for 1 minute, then reduce pace to MODERATE for 1 minute. Repeat 5 times.
- Finish last 15 minutes at MODERATE, gradually slowing to EASY.

THURSDAY

- Warm up for 5 minutes at EASY level.
- Increase to MODERATE for 10 minutes.
- Walk at CHALLENGING for 1 to 2 minutes (uphill, at 4 percent incline, or up stairs) then cool down by walking on flat surface for 1 to 2 minutes. Repeat once.
- Finish last 7 to 11 minutes at MODERATE.

SATURDAY

- Warm up for 5 minutes at EASY level.
- Increase to MODERATE for 5 minutes.
- Pick up pace to CHALLENGING for 5 minutes.
- Finish last 15 minutes at MODERATE.

SUNDAY

- Walk as slowly or quickly as you like for 30 minutes.

  Don't forget to warm up and cool down.

WEEKS 2 TO 4: REPEAT

IN OR OUT?

Here are a few things to consider before you decide where to take your walk.

INDOORS (treadmill)	OUTDOORS (sidewalk, trail, or road)
No ice, sleet, rain, snow, or darkness to worry about.	The sun in the sky, the wind in your hair, fresh air.
A nursery in a gym or a sleeping baby at home means you can squeeze in a workout when convenient.	You can bring the kids along; little ones can ride in carriers or all-terrain strollers.
Consistency, smooth surface; there's no stumbling on tree roots or cracked pavements.	Walking on an imperfect surface you burn slightly more calories (1 to 5 percent).
If you're visiting an unfamiliar area, you can play it safe and go to the hotel fitness center.	An excellent way to explore a new city—get a guidebook and take a walking tour.
Offers a super-controlled workout; you can precisely adjust the speed and incline.	Great variety of terrain; trekking up a hill can increase calorie burn, and since there is no way to flatten the incline, you're forced to push yourself.

Burn, Baby, Burn

Activity Step aerobics (with a 6- to 8-inch step)
Time 30 minutes

You Burn
284
CALORIES

*Based on a 140-pound woman.

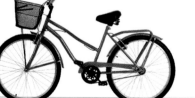

Drop

5 **DO IT NOW Get Fresh** Air, that is. People who **walked, hiked,** or **biked** on trails at least once a week were **twice as likely to get** 30 minutes of **exercise** almost **every day** as those who didn't head outdoors, University of Utah researchers found.

MYTH BUSTER

Fiction Wearing plastic pants or heavy sweats helps you burn more calories during a walk, run, or work-out at the gym.

Fact These pants *will* make you sweat a lot and the temporary water loss may show up on the scale, but quench your thirst and the "lost" pounds will magically reappear.

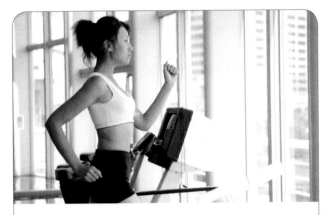

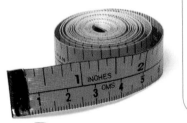

Speed Up Your Stride

Moderate exercise provides proven heart benefits, but you may have to speed up the pace to earn them. Studies have shown that, left to their own estimates of what's fast enough, many people aren't getting the fitness boost they think they are. To find the best speed, researchers from San Diego State University measured energy output as 97 people walked on a treadmill, then translated the participants' speeds to a formula everyone can use. **The right pace? About 100 steps a minute,** says lead researcher Simon J. Marshall, PhD. To load your iPod with songs that set the tempo, go to DjBPMStudio.com, click on "Index by BPM" (that's beats per minute), then choose 100. Check your pace with a pedometer. Or see "Listen to Lose" on page 206 for our Drop 5 Top 5 Exercise Song Picks.

Drop 5

DO IT NOW Pay Attention to More Than the Scale It isn't the *only* number to check. Before you start your plan, **take measurements** of your **hips, waist,** and **bust** so you have a baseline to track your progress. Measure the same spots (using the same tape measure) **once a week.** And pay attention to **how your clothes fit.** You can look forward to buying a new pair of skinny jeans down the road!

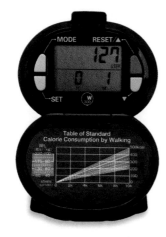

Count Your Steps

HERE'S THE THING ABOUT STEPS: THEY ADD UP.
And pedometers offer a lot of motivation. A
Stanford University review study confirmed it:
People who wear one take more than 2,000 extra
steps a day—that's about a mile!

**AN INACTIVE INDIVIDUAL, ON AVERAGE, TAKES
BETWEEN 1,000 AND 3,000 STEPS PER DAY.** If you
take 5,000 additional steps each day, you could
burn about 200 extra calories (this is an estimate—
your weight and the speed you walk both factor
in). Up it to 10,000 total steps on the weekend,
and you'll burn that much more. So strap on a
pedometer (pick one based on durability, accuracy,
performance, and ease of use) and start stepping!

**TAKE LONGISH STROLLS WITH YOUR SPOUSE,
CHILDREN, OR FRIENDS.** Walk the dog around
the block a few extra times. Use the stairs instead
of the elevator. Walk to your local grocery store,
church, post office, wherever. Walk every day, as
much as you can (see also "Diet Trap: Discounting
the Little Things" on page 126).

Learn from the "Losers"

"Think baby steps. When
I don't feel like walking,
I think, *I'll just put on my
shoes, anyway.* From there,
maybe I'll fool myself into
thinking, *I'm just going out
to check the weather—if
it's too cold or hot, I'll
come back in.* But once
I'm dressed and out the
door, I go!"

—KIM FRANCIS,
45 POUNDS LOST

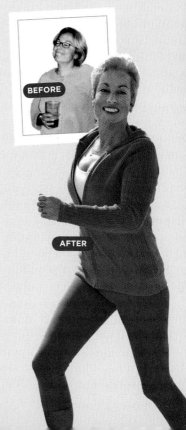

BEFORE

AFTER

GET
strong

When you strengthen your muscles, you're building a calorie-burning machine. In fact, some studies estimate that you burn an additional 35 to 40 calories per day with each pound of muscle you add to your body. The good news is there's no need to go to a gym—you can do our muscle-building plan at home!

The Drop

5 TWENTY-MINUTE MUSCLE-BUILDING PLAN

You can turn your home into a gym without buying any expensive equipment. Try these exercises three times a week, and you'll see weight-loss results in less than a month. You'll also develop lean muscle tissue, which burns more calories than fat does, even when you're just sitting in a chair.

WHAT YOU'LL NEED
Comfortable clothes to move in, a rubber ball about the size of a soccer ball, a bath towel, and a clear area to work out in.

WARM-UP
Before starting this workout, you should prepare for exercise with a 4-minute warm-up. To get your heart rate up, go to your staircase. Step up with your right foot, then up with the left; down with your right foot, down with the left. After 1 minute, switch and do 1 minute starting with the left foot. Repeat both sides. Step gently to protect your knees. If you don't have stairs, jog in place or walk briskly around the house.

AB TWIST

1. Sit on the floor (place a towel under you for comfort), feet shoulder width apart, knees up, toes pointing up so that you are resting on your heels. Holding the ball with both hands, extend your arms in front of you.

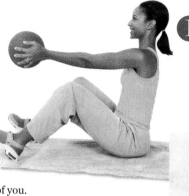

2. Slowly lie back, keeping abdominals tucked and tightened. Stop halfway to the floor and twist to the left, reaching toward the floor with the ball. Hold for a beat, then slowly twist to the right. Breathe normally and concentrate on contracting your abdominal muscles.

Number of reps 12 **Time** 2 minutes
Great for abdominals, glutes, hamstrings

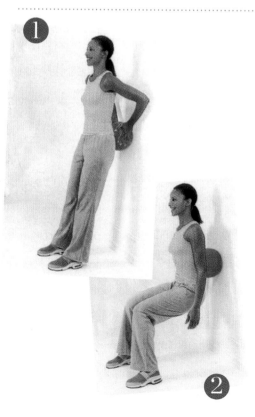

WALL SQUAT

1. Standing with your back to a bare wall, take the ball and place it in the small of your back just above your buttocks. Feet should be shoulder-width apart, toes forward, abdominals tucked.

2. Bend your knees to lower your body for five counts, until your hamstrings (the backs of your thighs) are almost parallel to the floor. Make sure your knees don't extend beyond your toes. Hold, then squeeze your glutes (your rear end) and press back up for five counts. Keep the ball between your back and the wall throughout the exercise.

Number of reps 12 **Time** 2 minutes
Great for glutes, hamstrings, quadriceps

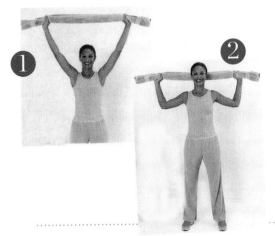

BACK PULL

1. Roll your towel lengthwise. Grasping an end in either hand, raise the towel over your head, arms extended.

2. Inhale, then slowly exhale, bending arms and lowering the towel down behind your head. Keep tension on the towel as you raise and lower it, but don't tense your neck.

Number of reps 12 **Time** 2 minutes
Great for back muscles

PUSH-UP

1. Fold your towel into a small square and place it under your knees for support. Kneeling on the towel, walk your hands forward until your torso is at a 45-degree incline to the floor. Hands should be slightly wider than shoulder width apart, with your fingers spread.

2. Tuck your abdominals as you lower yourself (keep your torso two inches off the floor). Hold, then squeeze your chest muscles as you press up to the starting position.

Number of reps 12 **Time** 2 minutes
Great for chest, arms

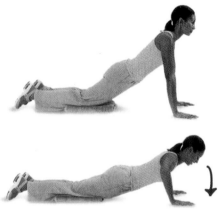

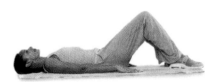

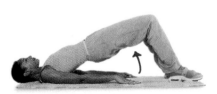

BRIDGE

1. Lie on your back, knees bent, feet flat on the floor, hands at your sides. (If you feel any tension in your neck, tuck your towel under your head for support.)

2. Inhale, then raise your bottom and your lower back off the floor as you exhale. Keep your back straight and your head and shoulders on the floor. Hold for one count. Slowly release and lower, but don't let your bottom touch the floor until you have completed all 12 repetitions. Focus on squeezing your glutes at the top of each rep.

Number of reps 12 **Time** 2 minutes
Great for abdominals, glutes, hamstrings

HAMSTRING CURL

1. Lie flat on your stomach with the ball between your ankles. Rest your head on your crossed arms. Squeezing the ball, lift your knees off the floor as high as you can, keeping your legs as straight as possible.

2. Slowly bend your knees until your feet point toward the ceiling. Exhale as you curl up; inhale as you release. Note: Keep your knees off the floor at all times. If you feel strain in your lower back, rest for a moment, then resume the exercise.

Number of reps 12 **Time** 2 minutes
Great for hamstrings, glutes, lower back

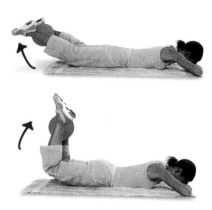

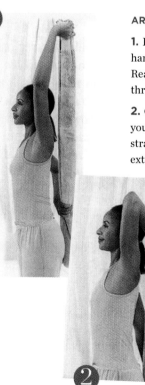

ARM EXTENSION

1. Roll the towel up lengthwise. Place one end in your left hand. Straighten your left arm directly over your head. Reach behind your back with your right arm and grasp three-quarters of the way down the towel.

2. Gently pull the towel down with your right arm, bending your left arm behind your head, so your elbow points straight up. Inhale, holding the towel steady. Exhale and extend your left arm back to starting position, keeping tension on the towel with your right arm. Do 12 repetitions. Switch hand positions, so right arm is extended overhead, and repeat.

Number of reps 12 on each side
Time 4 minutes
Great for triceps

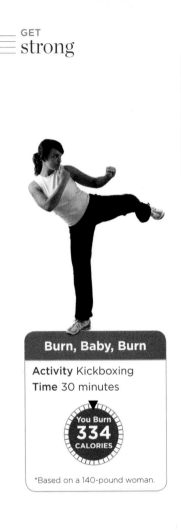

Whittle Your Middle

Starting in your mid-20s, tummy fat begins to creep on by a pound or two a year. But you can slow the spread with strength training. In a study at the University of Minnesota, overweight women who lifted weights just twice a week saw a much smaller increase in abdominal fat (7 percent) over a two-year period than women who didn't follow any particular exercise program (theirs went up 21 percent). While strength training may not take the place of a cardio workout, it's a great way to help keep belly fat at bay in only two workouts a week.

Burn, Baby, Burn

Activity Kickboxing
Time 30 minutes

You Burn
334
CALORIES

*Based on a 140-pound woman.

Drop

5 DO IT NOW **Prepare for Activity** Schedule exercise as seriously as work or social appointments (block out time in your calendar); **keep a bag of workout clothes,** shoes, and gear **in your office** or **car** so you are ready to work out **when time permits;** make inspiring **music playlists** (pages 190 and 206)—and keep your MP3 player charged and ready to go.

BEST FITNESS WEBSITES

The Good Housekeeping Research Institute examined 25 fitness sites, assessing experts' credentials, variety of workouts, price, and more. Here are our top three picks.

MyExercisePlan.com

STANDOUT FEATURE Self-customization. The site instructs you to choose two or three exercises for each muscle group from dozens of options—appealing if you're experienced at working out and just need a boost to restart.

OTHER PLUSES Easy navigation. The layout and step-by-step explanation pages were simple to use and follow.

CAVEATS With the onus on you to select your own plan, newbies might be daunted.

DeniseAustin.com

STANDOUT FEATURE Total-body integration. Austin is known for her fitness prowess, but this site also has sound diet and well-being advice (like menus and pep talks) to put you on track to a healthier body.

OTHER PLUSES Appealing charm. The site has a warm, inspiring voice that could really motivate the hesitant.

CAVEATS Many exercises require gear like a ball, weights, yoga mat, or bands.

MyHomePersonalTrainer.com

STANDOUT FEATURE Easily modified workouts. Drop-down menus let you select your exercise preferences, equipment, and free time; the site then creates a schedule with printable, illustrated routines.

OTHER PLUSES Individualized attention. Your personal trainer is accessible by e-mail for info and support.

CAVEATS The site's busy layout makes some features hard to find.

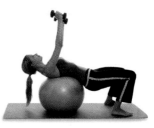

MYTH BUSTER
Fiction You can spot-reduce to lose weight. **Fact** On the contrary, the way to achieve sleeker legs or a flatter stomach, if that's where you're carrying your body fat, is to increase your lean muscle tissue throughout your body. By working all your muscles, you increase your metabolism. Up your metabolism and watch your eating, and you'll start looking the way you want to.

FUEL UP
with food

SMART SNACKS

PRE-WORKOUT You want something light and easy to digest, like a small handful of trail mix, a piece of fruit, a whole-grain fig bar, or one of our Smart Snacks, below. (If you've had a well-balanced meal within three hours of working out, you don't need a pre-exercise snack.)

These pre-workout munchies, recommended by Samantha B. Cassetty, MS, RD, nutrition director at the Good Housekeeping Research Institute, combine energizing carbs with muscle-boosting protein. None goes over 125 calories—so you can power your walks without putting on pounds.

Choose Well

Before exercise, fueling up with the right foods gives you energy so you can work harder. After exercise, eating right helps you recover faster and build more calorie-torching muscle—plus, you don't want to replace the calories you just burned by stopping at the drive-thru on the way home from the gym or reaching for the ice cream after playing tag with your kids. For best results, time your meals and snacks with your workouts.

- **Chocolaty Milk** For your sweet tooth—and stronger bones—down a bottle of Nesquik 100-calorie chocolate milk. Per serving: **100 CALORIES**

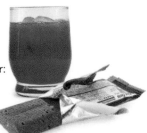

- **Bar Treat** Pick a snack bar with at least 3 grams of protein and no more than 100 calories. Wash it down with an OJ spritzer: Add ¼ cup juice to a large glass; fill with seltzer. Per serving: **125 CALORIES**

- **Mexican Cheese Melt** A spicy boost before an afternoon workout: Slice a whole-wheat tortilla in half; add a reduced-fat cheese stick to one side; heat in microwave 20 seconds; roll tortilla while warm, and dip into salsa. Per serving: **115 CALORIES**

POST-WORKOUT Here's where the fuel really matters. Within a few hours of your workout, you need a meal that includes carbohydrates, protein, and, yes, some fat, in order to speed muscle and tissue recovery. Research shows this is when muscles are able to soak up the most nutrients and when glycogen (your stored form of energy) is replaced most efficiently.

EMPTY-CALORIE EXERCISE CALCULATOR

Before you eat that cookie, brownie, or bag of chips, consider how long you'll have to work out to burn it off.

FOOD serving size, calories	TIME TO BURN IT OFF moderate walking*
Utz Regular Potato Chips 20 CHIPS, 150 CALORIES	**45** MINUTES
Cheetos 21 PIECES, 160 CALORIES	**48** MINUTES
Entenmann's Original Recipe Chocolate Chip Cookies 4 COOKIES, 190 CALORIES	**58** MINUTES
Mrs. Fields Semi-Sweet Chocolate Chip Cookie 210 CALORIES	**64** MINUTES
Hershey's Milk Chocolate Bar 210 CALORIES	**64** MINUTES
Oreo Cookies 4 COOKIES, 215 CALORIES	**65** MINUTES
Doritos 20 CHIPS, 270 CALORIES	**81** MINUTES
Snickers Candy Bar 280 CALORIES	**85** MINUTES
Krispy Kreme Glazed Raspberry Filled Doughnut 300 CALORIES	**91** MINUTES
Starbucks Blueberry Scone 460 CALORIES	**139** MINUTES
Ben & Jerry's Chocolate Fudge Brownie Ice Cream 1 CUP (ABOUT 1 SCOOP), 500 CALORIES	**156** MINUTES

*Calculations based on a 140-pound woman.

BEVERAGE EXERCISE CALCULATOR

Thinking of guzzling down a calorie-laden drink? First consider how long you'll have to exercise to work it off.

DRINK serving size, calories	TIME TO BURN IT OFF moderate walking*
Gatorade 16 OUNCES, 100 CALORIES	30 MINUTES
Lipton Iced Tea with Lemon 16 OUNCES, 120 CALORIES	36 MINUTES
Red Bull 8 OUNCES, 110 CALORIES	33 MINUTES
Wine 5 OUNCES, 120 CALORIES	36 MINUTES
Soda 12 OUNCES, 140 CALORIES	42 MINUTES
Beer 12 OUNCES, 150 CALORIES	45 MINUTES
Hawaiian Punch Fruit Juicy Red 16 OUNCES, 240 CALORIES	73 MINUTES
Starbucks Coffee Frappuccino 24 OUNCES, 330 CALORIES	100 MINUTES
Jamba Juice Banana Berry Smoothie 22 OUNCES, 400 CALORIES	121 MINUTES
McDonald's Chocolate Triple Thick Shake 21 OUNCES, 770 CALORIES	233 MINUTES

*Calculations based on a 140-pound woman.

FAST FOOD EXERCISE CALCULATOR

That fast-food meal or snack may be tempting, but consider how long you'll have to work out to burn it off.

FAST FOOD calories	TIME TO BURN IT OFF moderate walking*
Dunkin' Donuts Glazed Cake Donut 320 CALORIES	**96** MINUTES
McDonald's Medium French Fries 380 CALORIES	**115** MINUTES
2 slices Pizza Hut Cheese Pan Pizza 480 CALORIES	**145** MINUTES
KFC Extra-Crispy Chicken Breast 510 CALORIES	**154** MINUTES
Subway 6-Inch Tuna Sandwich 530 CALORIES	**160** MINUTES
Wendy's Baconater Single 610 CALORIES	**184** MINUTES
Sonic Drive-In Cheeseburger 630 CALORIES	**190** MINUTES
Burger King Whopper 670 CALORIES	**203** MINUTES
Arby's Market Fresh Roast Turkey & Swiss Sandwich 710 CALORIES	**213** MINUTES
Taco Bell Volcano Nachos 1,000 CALORIES	**303** MINUTES

*Calculations based on a 140-pound woman.

MORE FUN WAYS TO
up your fitness

Walking and weights aren't the only exercises that'll help you lose weight. For a relaxing change of pace, try a low-sweat workout, from ballet to Tai Chi. Or join a team and make your exercise a social event to help keep you motivated. If you're busy, you can burn an extra 100 calories here and there—fun activities like playing catch with your kids for 35 minutes or chores like weeding the garden for 20 minutes will do the trick!

Low-Sweat Workouts

If you want to get in shape but you're not up for a marathon, try some of these less-taxing alternatives.

PILATES

Named after Joseph Pilates (pronounced puh-*lah*-tees), who developed a set of floor exercises 70 years ago, this workout combines strength, flexibility, balance, core strengthening, and control training with resistance exercises. It's done individually or in groups, with or without specific pieces of specially designed equipment. A workout lasts 45 to 90 minutes, and although it's not aerobic at lower levels, advanced students can get cardiovascular benefit.

You burn 168 calories per 1-hour session

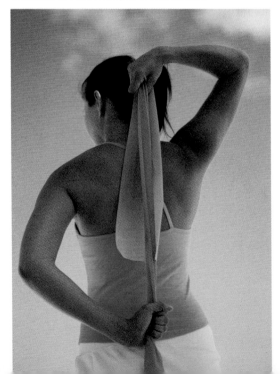

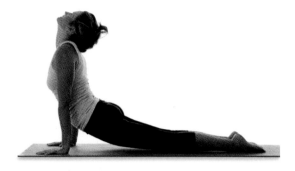

WATER WORKOUTS

Exercising in water is increasingly popular with people who have been injured by high-impact workouts. Participants can walk on underwater treadmills or perform arm, leg, and abdominal exercises. Minute for minute, it burns fewer calories than the same exercises performed on land, but many people find they can train longer, in part because water pressure helps blood circulate so that the heart doesn't have to work as hard.

You burn 270 calories per 1-hour session

TAI CHI

This ancient Chinese practice improves strength, flexibility, concentration, and balance by combining mental discipline with physical movement. When done correctly, Tai Chi can raise your heart rate to 60 percent of maximum, qualifying as moderate exercise. Thighs and hips do much of the work, just as in high-impact aerobics—but without the jumping. And it just may keep you young: Aerobic capacity, a measure of how the heart, lungs, and circulatory system are working, declines with age, but one study demonstrated that Tai Chi practitioners managed to slow the process through regular practice.

You burn 270 calories per 1-hour session

YOGA

Now practiced by more than 4 million Americans, yoga improves flexibility, muscle strength, and endurance. It consists of deep-breathing exercises and postures or poses. Yoga also involves muscle toning and some aerobic movement. The poses can be adapted to any fitness level. As you increase the depth of practice, the benefits increase. It's best to start with a supervised class, so you learn how to do the positions correctly; otherwise, you risk injury and may not get the full effect.

You burn 200 calories per 1-hour session

BALLET

You don't have to be a little girl with dreams of becoming a prima ballerina: This graceful, exacting form of dance is becoming a popular way for adults to stretch and strengthen underused muscles and improve balance, flexibility, and coordination. An added benefit is improved posture: Ballet moves teach you to align your body and promote fitness discipline.

You burn 320 calories per 1-hour session

All calorie burn-off calculations based on a 140-pound woman.

EASIEST WAYS TO BURN 100 CALORIES

Ready to Drop 5 faster? Figure out how much time you have, then choose any one of these activities.*

10 MINUTES

Run around the block.

Jump rope quickly.

Work out to a step aerobics video.

Vacuum the rugs.

Mop the bathrooms or kitchen.

Row a boat at the park.

Engage a friend in a serious Ping-Pong match.

15 MINUTES

Climb up and down your stairs at a moderate pace.

Play touch football with the family.

Swim laps, any style, at a leisurely pace.

Go roller-skating.

Sled in the park with the kids.

Hit some tennis balls.

20 MINUTES

Power walk (walking at a brisk pace while pumping the arms).

Shoot hoops with your teens.

Weed the garden.

Turn up the music and dance around the room.

25 MINUTES

Rake the lawn and sack the leaves.

Bike around the neighborhood at a leisurely speed.

Go horseback riding.

30 MINUTES

Throw a Frisbee around.

Go ballroom dancing.

Lift light weights.

Wash your car.

Sweep the floors.

35 MINUTES

Dust the house.

Practice the piano or violin.

Set the table and prepare a meal.

Play catch with your kids.

Clear the table and wash the pots, pans, and dishes.

40 MINUTES

Iron your clothes.

Window-shop.

Unload the dryer and fold the laundry.

Cruise the supermarket aisles.

*Calorie burn-off calculations based on a 140-pound woman.

Stand Up to Slim Down

Here's an easy way to burn twice as many calories: Just stand up. In a series of studies on the physiological differences between sitting and standing, researchers at the University of Missouri–Columbia found that standing doubles your metabolic rate because you need more strength to hold up your body. It also helps muscles siphon fat out of the bloodstream. So stay on your feet: Try ironing while watching TV or use a chalkboard for to-do lists.

MYTH BUSTER

Fiction Early morning is the best time to exercise. **Fact** "The best time to exercise is anytime you can do it," says Samantha B. Cassetty, MS, RD. "You get the same payoffs and burn essentially the same number of calories whenever you work out. What's important is doing it regularly."

Some studies have shown that first-thing-in-the-morning exercisers are more likely to stick with a regimen than those who start late in the day, but that's because it's probably easier to postpone an evening workout until tomorrow. So whether you have more time or energy in the morning, afternoon, or at night, the important thing is that you do it.

Learn from the "Losers"

"My exercise-more tip: Get some serious workout clothes. Having pretty fitness wear got me excited about going to the gym."

—SARAH BELL,
120 POUNDS LOST

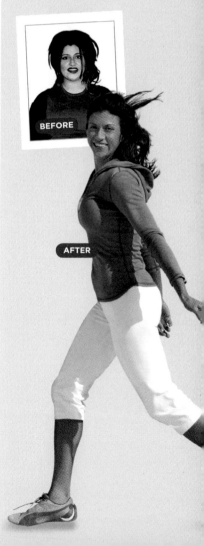

BEFORE

AFTER

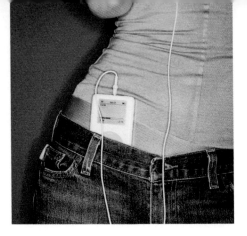

The Dream Team

To stay motivated, join a team for, say, volleyball, bowling, soccer, or basketball. According to researchers from the University of Copenhagen in Denmark, women involved in team sports may have a fitness advantage. Those who took up soccer were more likely to continue after the 16-week study ended, compared to women who started running (a solo activity). The players were motivated by the social interaction.

LISTEN TO LOSE

People who work out to music could lose twice as much as those who exercise in silence, suggests recent research, because music helps you stick to your workout so you stay at it longer. Make your next exercise session really sing with the *Good Housekeeping* editors' Drop 5 Top 5 Exercise Song Picks. (We've included the beats per minute, since experts recommend walking at a rate of at least 100 steps per minute to maximize benefits.)

1. **"VIVA LA VIDA"** (138 b.p.m.), Coldplay

2. **"CITY OF BLINDING LIGHTS"** (139 b.p.m.), U2

3. **"SOAK UP THE SUN"** (120 b.p.m.), Sheryl Crow

4. **"AMERICAN GIRL"** (114 b.p.m.), Tom Petty and the Heartbreakers

5. **"RAY OF LIGHT"** (127 b.p.m.), Madonna

Drop
5
DO IT NOW Laugh More Often It's no joke: **A study** from Vanderbilt University showed that **you can burn up to 40 calories by laughing** genuinely for **10 to 15 minutes.**

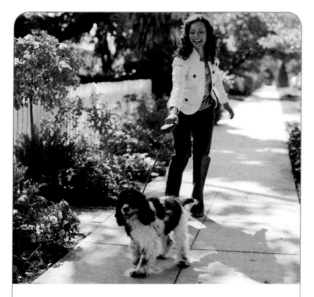

Get Fit with Fido

The most effective personal trainers may be furry and four-legged. Researchers from the University of Victoria in British Columbia found that people who own dogs walk almost twice as much as those who don't. One key reason: Even when pet owners are feeling lazy, they will head outdoors to give their little buddy a chance to relieve himself and get some exercise.

MYTH BUSTER

Fiction Your body won't burn fat unless you exercise for more than 20 minutes. **Fact** You burn fat around the clock, whether you're exercising or not. For the biggest calorie burn, exercise as hard as you comfortably can (you should still be able to carry on a conversation) for as long as you can.

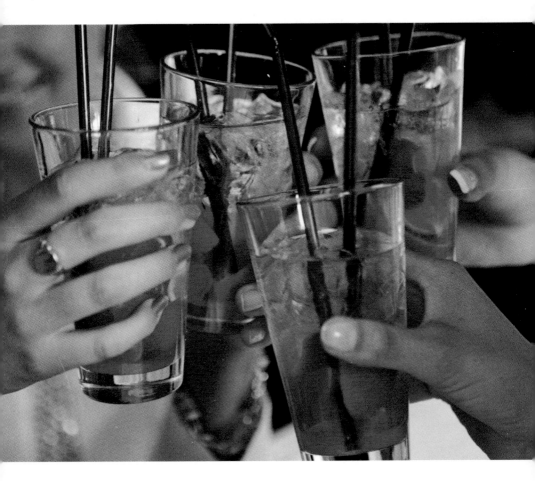

SWEET CELEBRATIONS
handling
holidays
& parties

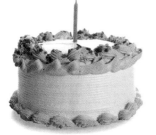

You can celebrate good times without derailing your diet. Here, how to eat, drink, and enjoy a slice of cake—without packing on the pounds.

PARTY TIME OFTEN TRANSLATES into eating time. In fact, celebrations are usually coupled with special foods—turkey with stuffing and pumpkin pie at Thanksgiving, caviar and champagne on New Year's, latkes for Hanukkah—not to mention your grandmother's special shortbread cookies at Christmas! Merrymaking means special, often rich, food—and reasons to share and indulge in them. And according to a study from the National Institutes of Health, the fabled holiday season weight gain (from Thanksgiving to New Year's) is no myth. While the pounds added were modest (about one each year), that weight tends to stay on and accumulate over time. And it doesn't even include weight gain from excess calories scarfed down at Fourth of July barbecues and your children's birthday parties. Yet it's hard to munch on carrots when everyone else is enjoying canapés or cake. In order to enjoy celebrations and fit into that party dress for the next big event, you need to have a plan.

Try the Drop 5 Top 5 tactics for holidays and parties—and any other special events with tempting treats.

Drop
5
Top 5
SWEET CELEBRATION TIPS

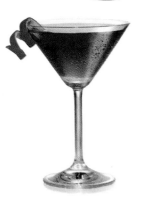

Partiers beware: The more you drink, the less aware you'll be of how much you are consuming. Have just one fancy cocktail—and enjoy it.

1 **BE PREPARED** Before that birthday picnic, holiday dinner, or family get-together, recognize the situations that cause you to overindulge, then strategize. "When it comes to eating behavior, mental rehearsal helps you anticipate cues and build the skills necessary to respond to them," says David Kessler, MD, author of *The End of Overeating*. "It only takes a minute or two to rehearse your performance, preferably just before you enter the high-risk environment in which you'll likely be cued." Then, you'll know your line of attack (have just a small piece of cake and only one cocktail, for example) when you enter the dieting danger zone.

2 **BE A PICKY EATER** Think of the calories you'll eat as money in the bank. Make wise investments with your calories, selecting the best of the offerings and passing up foods that are available anytime. (Aunt Moira's world-famous latkes are worth every calorie; a bowl of potato chips is not.) Pick your favorite special foods to splurge on and eat one or two, not the entire tray.

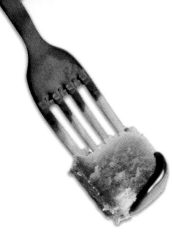

Don't play the blame game if you eat more cake, say, than you intended; use your remorse to redouble your dieting efforts.

3 **KEEP MOVING** Exercise burns calories and helps you control your weight—but only if you work out on a regular basis. During the holidays and while on vacation, it's tempting to abandon your exercise routine, but in truth, this is the worst time to skimp. Every week, try to have as many "normal" days—when you eat healthy foods and exercise—as possible. "Challenge yourself to figure out exactly when you can squeeze in exercise on the busiest day of the week," says certified strength and conditioning specialist Myatt Murphy. "If you can make the hardest day doable, you'll be surprised how easily you'll find time to exercise during the rest of the week."

If it's just impossible to take an exercise break, then think of other ways you can be active. "Even if you're not challenging your body with your usual workout, there are other ways to burn a few extra calories," says Murphy. If you're at a party, volunteer to clear the tables or fetch items from the kitchen; if you're at a family gathering, take twenty minutes to play tag with your nieces and nephews; on vacation, go for walks.

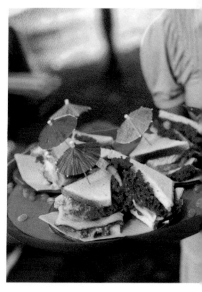

Don't Go Shopping Hungry

Set up your holiday shopping schedule so you hit the mall with a full stomach; the last thing you need is to graze your way from store to store. Or carry a small, calorie-controlled snack with you. For example, choose a 100-calorie granola bar (or see pages 52–55 and 121 for additional suggestions) instead of a 730-calorie Cinnabon roll.

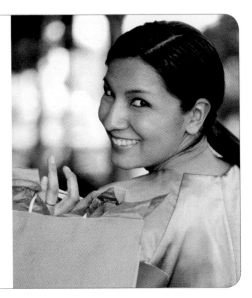

DAILY CALORIE TARGETS

Consult these guidelines as you choose
recipes, meals, and snacks from this chapter.

FOR WOMEN		FOR MEN	
Breakfast	350	Breakfast	450
Lunch	500	Lunch	600
Dinner	500	Dinner	600
Snack	100	Snack	200
Optional Treat	100	Optional Treat	200
TOTAL	1,450–1,550	Total	1,850–2,050

If you go a little over (or under) at any meal, compensate by adjusting your calories later in the day. Have the optional treat once a day, or save up those calories and have a larger treat every other day, or even two larger 350-calorie treats a couple of days a week. If you want to cut calories a bit more, you can also skip the optional treat altogether.

4 BE AT PEACE WITH YOUR CRAVINGS

A Drexel University study found that people who'd been taught to use techniques similar to mindfulness meditation (accepting that thoughts are just thoughts and don't require a rush to judgment or action) were better able to resist a treat—in this case, a package of Hershey's Kisses—than those who didn't have the training. "If you try to make your cravings go away, all your focus is on the food," says researcher Evan Forman, PhD. "But if you just exist with the thought, it loses its power." One way to make that easier: Take a moment to think about what you want out of life that feeding your craving might deny you. To be fit enough to hike with your kids? Slim enough to wear a slinky red dress to your New Year's Eve party? "Identifying what's ultimately important to you will allow that goal—rather than a food craving—to direct your behavior," says Forman.

5 DROP THE ALL-OR-NOTHING ATTITUDE

"I blew it at lunch, so I may as well pig out at dinner." All right, you had a celebratory lunch with a few friends. Or maybe you drank three jumbo-size margaritas at a Cinco de Mayo party or ordered an appetizer and shared a dessert on a special evening out. All told, you've taken in an extra 500 to 600 calories for the day. If you then take a no-holds-barred approach to your next meal, you risk turning that 500- to 600-calorie infraction into a 1,500- to 1,600-calorie debacle. Don't beat yourself up: If you do overindulge, acknowledge that you feel bad about it, but use that energy to redouble your efforts— shift your mind-set from "I am a colossal screwup" to "I'm back in the game!"

Hold Back at the Buffet

Don't rush to the head of the line! If you're first to get your food at the buffet, you'll be finished eating before the rest of the party and tempted to head back to fill your plate with more food. Also, choose to chat away from the food table so you're not tempted to consume absentmindedly.

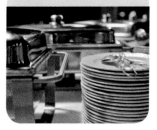

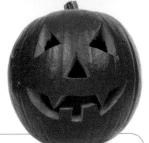

AVOID HOLIDAY
weight gain

The stretch from Halloween right up until the beginning of January is jam-packed with festivities, fun—and lots of diet temptations. This year is going to be different, though. You're going to start the New Year fitting into your slimmest slacks by following these very simple, doable tips and tricks during the holiday season.

Terrifying Treats

Looking for some incentive to stop at just one or two fun-size candies? Take a look at how fast the numbers add up:

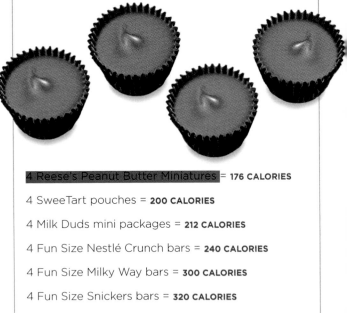

4 Reese's Peanut Butter Miniatures = 176 **CALORIES**

4 SweeTart pouches = **200 CALORIES**

4 Milk Duds mini packages = 212 **CALORIES**

4 Fun Size Nestlé Crunch bars = **240 CALORIES**

4 Fun Size Milky Way bars = **300 CALORIES**

4 Fun Size Snickers bars = **320 CALORIES**

4 Fun Size Butterfinger bars = **400 CALORIES**

Drop

5

DO IT NOW Track Your Wrappers To prevent yourself from mindlessly munching through half a dozen bite-size treats, **count** your **empty wrappers.** This will help you keep a **tally of your intake** and remind you to **stop snacking.**

HALLOWEEN HELP

"It is easy to get enticed by those bite-size candies. But one usually turns into more, and before you know it, you have eaten the equivalent of a full-size candy bar," says Tara Gidus, MS, RD, a spokeswoman for the American Dietetic Association. Pick your Halloween treats with your calorie bottom line in mind.

DIET MADNESS	DIET MAKEOVER	YOU SAVE
Hershey's Milk Chocolate Snack Size Bar 77 CALORIES	2 Tootsie Roll Midgees 47 CALORIES	**30** CALORIES
Skittles Fun Size 80 CALORIES	2 Smarties Candy Rolls 50 CALORIES	**30** CALORIES
M&M's Fun Size 90 CALORIES	2 Rolo Caramels 55 CALORIES	**35** CALORIES
Butterfinger Fun Size 85 CALORIES	2 Hershey's Kisses filled with peanut butter 49 CALORIES	**36** CALORIES
2 Charms Blow Pops 120 CALORIES	2 Dum Dum Pops 51 CALORIES	**69** CALORIES

Deal with Seasonal Stress

It's easy to underestimate the toll the holidays take—physically, psychologically, and emotionally. You may be feeling financially pinched or extra tired from lack of sleep. And extended visits with your family are not always tension-free. To avoid using eating as an emotional crutch, try these strategies for basic self-preservation.

- **TAKE A QUICK WALK** A California State University study that tracked frequent emotional snackers found that those who went for a brisk five-minute walk when they felt frazzled were much less likely to eat than those who just sat still.

- **DON'T GET CAUGHT UP IN THE HOLIDAY FRENZY** If there are too many parties, decline a few. If all the shopping stress is causing you to overeat, talk to your family about ways to make this year less chaotic. The more open and honest you are with yourself and with family and friends, the less likely it is that you'll turn to food to soothe yourself during the season.

- **BUDDY UP TO MANAGE STRESS** To avoid gaining weight now, you need commitment and awareness. It's best to work on both with a group of people—or even one or two close friends—whom you can call when an emotionally triggered eating craving strikes. So instead of polishing off a carton of ice cream after a stressful family dinner, phone a friend to share how you feel and deal with the emotions (see "Emotional Eating 101" on page 71).

Crunch Time

Holiday shopping may trim your wallet, but it could also flatten your belly. As you search store shelves, stand tall and squeeze your stomach muscles for five seconds (pretend you're bracing yourself to lift a heavy box). Tada! You've done the equivalent of one sit-up, says exercise physiologist Pete McCall, MS, of the American Council on Exercise.

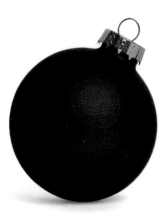

Write It Down

You've already learned in Eating In (page 64) about the importance of keeping a food and exercise diary. This is even more crucial during the holidays, when you'll be tempted with foods you might not normally eat (baking twelve dozen sugar cookies on a random Sunday would be crazy, but at Christmastime, it's practically required). Research has shown that writing everything down is the one thing—more than anything else—that helps successful dieters lose weight and keep it off. It's the willingness to pay attention to what you're eating that's critical.

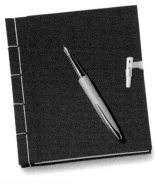

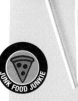

MAKE IT A HABIT
Pass Out Candy You Don't Love

If you buy treats that aren't your all-time faves, you'll be less likely to overindulge. For most adults, gummies, sour candies, and other nonchocolate sweets are easier to resist. Also, wait until the last minute to buy candy. The less time it spends in your house, the smaller your chance for temptation.

DO THE MATH

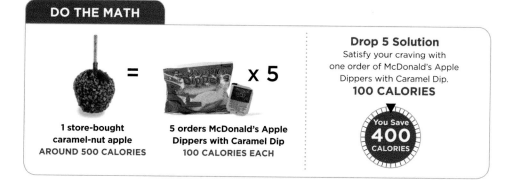

= x 5

1 store-bought caramel-nut apple
AROUND 500 CALORIES

5 orders McDonald's Apple Dippers with Caramel Dip
100 CALORIES EACH

Drop 5 Solution
Satisfy your craving with one order of McDonald's Apple Dippers with Caramel Dip.
100 CALORIES

You Save **400** CALORIES

HEALTHY RECIPE MAKEOVER
Holiday Herb-Roasted Potatoes

Classic holiday scalloped potatoes
SINGLE SERVING: 295 CALORIES
Healthy Makeover
Holiday Herb-Roasted Potatoes
SINGLE SERVING: 125 CALORIES

You Save
170
CALORIES

No need to drown your spuds in cheese and butter: This is a light alternative to traditional high-fat, creamy potato side dishes.

Active time 15 minutes
Total time 45 minutes
Makes 6 side-dish servings

- 2 **tablespoons margarine or butter**
- 1 **tablespoon chopped fresh parsley**
- ½ **teaspoon freshly grated lemon peel**
- ½ **teaspoon salt**
- ⅛ **teaspoon coarsely ground black pepper**
- 1½ **pounds small red potatoes, cut in half**

1. Preheat oven to 450°F. In 3-quart saucepan, melt margarine with parsley, lemon peel, salt, and pepper over medium-low heat. Remove saucepan from heat; add potatoes and toss well to coat.

2. Place potato mixture in center of 24" by 18" sheet of heavy-duty aluminum foil. Fold edges over and pinch to seal tightly.

3. Place package in jelly-roll pan and bake until potatoes are tender when they are pierced (through foil) with knife, about 30 minutes.

EACH SERVING: ABOUT 125 CALORIES, 2 G PROTEIN, 20 G CARBOHYDRATE, 4 G TOTAL FAT (2 G SATURATED), 10 MG CHOLESTEROL, 241 MG SODIUM, 2 G FIBER

MAKE SIMPLE SUBSTITUTIONS
(and Drop Close to 1,000 Calories from Your Holiday Meals)

Use this tactic on favorite holiday dishes, and you can save loads of calories. Substitute nonfat milk for whole, nonfat half-and-half for heavy cream in soups and bisques, and nonfat sour cream for full-fat in calorie-laden dips. Try low-fat broth instead of fat-based mixtures for basting meats. Choose light meat over dark. Here, our slimmed-down versions of some seasonal classics.

DIET MADNESS	DIET MAKEOVER	YOU SAVE
Green bean casserole 148 CALORIES PER 1 CUP	Lean Green Bean Casserole 95 CALORIES PER 1 CUP See recipe on page 221	**53** CALORIES
Traditional latkes 150 CALORIES PER LATKE	Light Latkes 65 CALORIES PER LATKE See recipe on page 226	**85** CALORIES
Bread crumb stuffing 176 CALORIES PER 1/2 CUP	Vegetable-Herb Stuffing 90 CALORIES PER 1/2 CUP See recipe on page 223	**86** CALORIES
Brownies 206 CALORIES PER BAR	Lighter Brownies 95 CALORIES PER BAR See recipe on page 213	**111** CALORIES
Scalloped potatoes 295 CALORIES PER SERVING	Holiday Herb-Roasted Potatoes 130 CALORIES PER SERVING See recipe, opposite	**165** CALORIES
Pumpkin pie 316 CALORIES PER SLICE	Pumpkin Spice Ring 110 CALORIES PER SLICE See recipe on page 224	**206** CALORIES
Classic eggnog 440 CALORIES PER 1/2 CUP	Light and Creamy Eggnog 105 CALORIES PER 1/2 CUP See recipe on page 229	**335** CALORIES

Put Holiday Side Dishes on a Diet

Try enjoying the autumn harvest simply prepared, without lots of extra fat and sugar. A whole baked sweet potato, for example, is delicious with just a sprinkle of cinnamon or nutmeg (around 100 calories), so skip the butter, brown sugar, nuts, and marshmallows dressing up the usual sweet potato casserole (around 250 calories per ½ cup serving). For a list of weight-reducing holiday recipe swaps, see page 219.

DIET TRAP
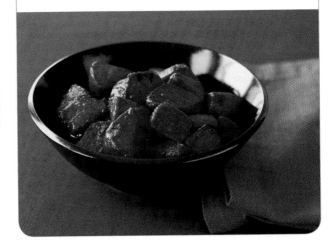

Waiting Until January 1 to Change Your Eating Habits

Committing to a "diet" in the future encourages you to binge in the here and now. And you'll go crazy with high-cal foods because you anticipate giving them up. Be mindful now, and you won't have to dig yourself out of a two-month glut.

Drop

5 **DO IT NOW Carry a Sprig of Mint During the Holidays** A whiff of **peppermint** may help you **shed pounds,** according to a study at Wheeling Jesuit University in West Virginia. Investigators tracked twenty-seven adults for two five-day periods and found that those **who wafted peppermint oil** under their nose every two hours ate almost 350 fewer calories a day than the nonsniffers. The aroma **increases alertness,** so you're less likely to snack out of fatigue or boredom, say the authors. Chewing mint leaves or a stick of mint-flavored gum may also do the trick.

Lean Green Bean Casserole

About 30 million households will serve this dish on Thanksgiving. Too bad it's not as good for you as it tastes. We switched to low-fat milk and reduced-sodium broth, and traded canned french-fried onions for oven-fried ones, trimming the total fat by 8 grams and dropping the sodium by 257 milligrams. Seconds, anyone?

Active time 30 minutes
Total time 45 minutes
Makes 8 side-dish servings

- Olive-oil nonstick cooking spray
- 1 large onion (12 ounces), cut into ½-inch-thick slices and separated into rings
- 5 tablespoons all-purpose flour
- ⅜ teaspoon salt
- 1½ pounds green beans, trimmed
- 1 tablespoon butter or trans-fat-free margarine
- 1 large shallot, finely chopped
- 1 container (10 ounces) sliced cremini or white mushrooms
- ¼ teaspoon ground black pepper
- 1 cup reduced-sodium chicken broth
- ½ cup low-fat (1%) milk

1. Preheat oven to 425°F. Line large cookie sheet with foil; spray with nonstick spray. In bowl, toss onion with 2 tablespoons flour and ⅛ teaspoon salt. Spread onion in single layer on prepared foil; spray onion with nonstick spray. Bake 14 minutes; toss to rearrange, then spray again. Bake 15 minutes or until crisp.

2. Meanwhile, in 5-quart saucepot, heat *3 quarts water* to boiling on high. Add beans and cook, uncovered, 5 minutes or until tender-crisp. Drain beans in colander; rinse under cold water. Drain.

3. In 4-quart saucepan, melt butter on medium. Add shallot; cook 2 minutes, stirring. Add mushrooms; cook 7 to 8 minutes or until tender, stirring often. Stir in remaining ¼ teaspoon salt, ¼ teaspoon pepper, and remaining 3 tablespoons flour; cook 1 minute. Add broth and milk; heat to boiling on high,

stirring. Reduce heat to low; cook 2 minutes. Add beans.

4. Transfer mixture to 2-quart baking dish; bake 15 minutes. Stir mixture; top with onion. Bake 5 minutes or until sauce is bubbly.

EACH 1-CUP SERVING: ABOUT 95 CALORIES, 5 G PROTEIN, 16 G CARBOHYDRATE, 2 G TOTAL FAT (0 G SATURATED), 1 MG CHOLESTEROL, 285 MG SODIUM, 4 G FIBER

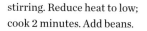

Classic green bean casserole
SINGLE SERVING: 148 CALORIES
Healthy Makeover Lean Green Bean Casserole
SINGLE SERVING: 95 CALORIES

You Save
53
CALORIES

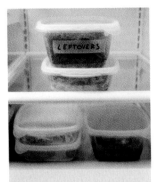

MAKE IT A HABIT
Don't Hoard
Leftovers

When you host the holiday meal, keep only the meat, baked sweet potatoes, veggies, and salad. Be sure to send all the high-calorie goodies home with guests. Or pack a few individual servings of the calorie-rich fare for your family.

TURKEY SANDWICH: FOUL PLAY?

For some people, the classic day-after-Thanksgiving sandwich is the reason to cook the turkey in the first place. But when you see just how much you are gobbling up, you may punt the traditional version and go for the trimmed one (saving 555 calories!).

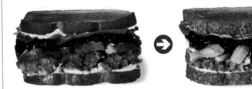

CLASSIC SANDWICH	SLIMMER SANDWICH
2 slices Pepperidge Farm Farmhouse Hearty White Bread **240 CALORIES**	2 slices Pepperidge Farm Light Style Soft Wheat Bread **90 CALORIES**
4 ounces light and dark turkey with skin **194 CALORIES**	4 ounces skinless breast meat **153 CALORIES**
½ cup canned sweetened cranberry sauce **210 CALORIES**	¼ cup canned sweetened cranberry sauce **105 CALORIES**
½ cup prepared bread stuffing **176 CALORIES**	¼ cup prepared bread stuffing **88 CALORIES**
1 large leaf romaine lettuce **5 CALORIES**	1 large leaf romaine lettuce **5 CALORIES**
2 tablespoons mayonnaise **206 CALORIES**	1 tablespoon light mayonnaise **35 CALORIES**
Total: **1,031** calories	Total: **476** calories

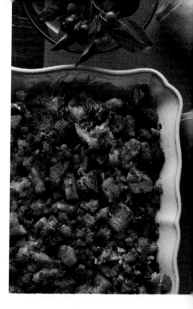

HEALTHY RECIPE MAKEOVER
Vegetable-Herb Stuffing

At 86 fewer calories and 4 grams less fat per serving than classic bread stuffing, this recipe is a win-win. The secret? We replaced the butter with olive oil and increased the ratio of veggies and herbs to bread.

Active time 25 minutes
Total time 1 hour 25 minutes
Makes 12 cups or 24 servings

- 1½ **loaves (16 ounces each) sliced firm white bread**
- 1 **tablespoon olive oil**
- 2 **medium carrots, finely chopped**
- 2 **medium stalks celery, finely chopped**
- 1 **medium onion, finely chopped**
- ½ **cup loosely packed fresh parsley leaves, coarsely chopped**
- ¾ **teaspoon poultry seasoning**
- ½ **teaspoon salt**
- ¼ **teaspoon freshly ground black pepper**
- 2½ **cups chicken broth**

1. Preheat oven to 400°F. Grease shallow 3- or 3½-quart ceramic or glass baking dish; set aside. Arrange bread on 2 large ungreased cookie sheets, and toast in oven 16 to 17 minutes or until golden and dry, turning slices over halfway through toasting.

2. Meanwhile, in a 12-inch nonstick skillet, heat oil on medium 1 minute. Add carrots, celery, and onion, and cook about 12 minutes or until vegetables are tender and lightly browned, stirring occasionally. Remove skillet from heat; stir in parsley, poultry seasoning, salt, and pepper.

3. With serrated knife, cut bread into ½-inch cubes, and place in very large bowl. Reset oven control to 325°F. Add chicken broth and vegetable mixture to bread in bowl; toss until bread mixture is evenly moistened.

4. Spoon stuffing into prepared baking dish. Cover dish with foil and bake stuffing 30 minutes. Remove foil and bake 15 to 20 minutes longer or until heated through and lightly browned on top.

EACH ½-CUP SERVING: ABOUT 90 CALORIES, 3 G PROTEIN, 16 G CARBOHYDRATE, 2 G TOTAL FAT (0 G SATURATED), 0 MG CHOLESTEROL, 270 MG SODIUM, 1 G FIBER

Bread crumb stuffing
SINGLE SERVING: 176 CALORIES
Healthy Makeover Vegetable-Herb Stuffing
SINGLE SERVING: 90 CALORIES

You Save **86** CALORIES

HEALTHY RECIPE MAKEOVER
Pumpkin Spice Ring

This is a delicious dessert that saves tons of calories and fat when compared to the traditional Thanksgiving favorite, pumpkin pie.

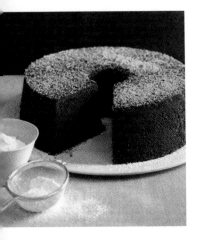

Active time 25 minutes
Total time 1 hour
Makes 16 servings

- 1¼ **cups cake flour (not self-rising)**
- 1 **teaspoon ground cinnamon**
- ¾ **teaspoon salt**
- ½ **teaspoon ground ginger**
- ¼ **teaspoon grated nutmeg**
- 2 **cups confectioners' sugar, plus additional for sprinkling**
- 1⅔ **cups (12 to 14 large) egg whites**
- 1½ **teaspoons cream of tartar**
- 1½ **teaspoons vanilla extract**
- 1 **cup (half a 15-ounce can) pure pumpkin (not pumpkin-pie mix)**

1. Preheat oven to 375°F. In medium bowl, with fork, mix flour, cinnamon, salt, ginger, nutmeg, and 1 cup confectioners' sugar; set aside.

2. In large bowl, with mixer at high speed, beat egg whites and cream of tartar until soft peaks form; beat in vanilla. Beating at high speed, sprinkle in remaining 1 cup confectioners' sugar, 2 tablespoons at a time, beating until sugar dissolves and whites stand in stiff peaks. Remove 1 cup beaten egg-white mixture to medium bowl; fold in pumpkin.

3. With rubber spatula or wire whisk, fold flour mixture into beaten egg whites in large bowl just until flour disappears. Then, gently fold in pumpkin mixture. Do not overmix.

4. Pour batter into ungreased 10-inch tube pan. Bake 35 minutes or until cake springs back when lightly touched. Invert pan with cake still inside onto funnel or bottle; cool cake completely in pan.

5. Loosen cake from pan; place on cake plate. Sprinkle with confectioners' sugar.

EACH SERVING: ABOUT 110 CALORIES, 4 G PROTEIN, 23 G CARBOHYDRATE, 0 G TOTAL FAT (0 G SATURATED), 0 MG CHOLESTEROL, 154 MG SODIUM, 1 G FIBER

Pumpkin pie
SINGLE SERVING: 316 CALORIES
**Healthy Makeover
Pumpkin Spice Ring**
SINGLE SERVING: 110 CALORIES

You Save
206
CALORIES

Some slices are more diet-defying than others. (All calorie counts are for one-eighth of a nine-inch, single-crust pie.)

PIE	CALORIES
Chocolate cream	522
Pecan	503
Mince	477
Apple	411
Banana cream	387
Sweet potato	363
Lemon meringue	362
Pumpkin	316

PDA Party Help

Need more help navigating that table of temptation, a.k.a. the buffet? Use your personal digital assistant (PDA). Just go to Calorieking.com/mobile, type in the treat that's threatening your willpower (the database is filled with nutrition info for more than 50,000 foods), and click "go." You'll know within seconds how many calories are in that slice of chocolate cake.

DO THE MATH

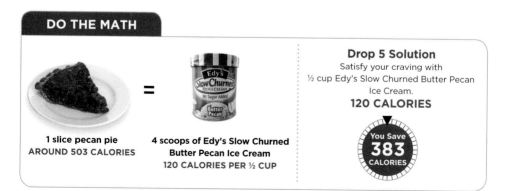

1 slice pecan pie
AROUND 503 CALORIES

=

4 scoops of Edy's Slow Churned Butter Pecan Ice Cream
120 CALORIES PER ½ CUP

Drop 5 Solution
Satisfy your craving with ½ cup Edy's Slow Churned Butter Pecan Ice Cream.
120 CALORIES

You Save
383
CALORIES

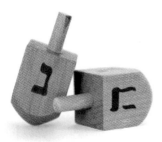

HEALTHY RECIPE MAKEOVER
Light Latkes

 Potato latkes are a Hanukkah tradition, since they're cooked in oil, the sacred fuel central to the story of the menorah's lighting. Alas, that oil adds to the fat and calories in these crispy patties. This year, try our lighter twist, which we baked instead.

Active time 20 minutes
Total time 50 minutes
Makes 12 latkes

    Canola-oil nonstick
    cooking spray
2   large egg whites
3   tablespoons snipped fresh
    chives
2   tablespoons all-purpose
    flour
1   tablespoon fresh lemon juice
¾   teaspoon salt
¼   teaspoon ground black
    pepper
2½ pounds baking (russet)
    potatoes (4 medium), peeled
    Applesauce (optional)

1. Preheat oven to 450°F. Spray very large cookie sheet (20″ by 14″) or 2 smaller ones with canola-oil nonstick cooking spray.

2. In large bowl, with fork, mix egg whites, chives, flour, lemon juice, salt, and pepper. In food processor with shredding disk attached, or on coarse side of box grater, shred potatoes. Place potatoes in colander in sink; squeeze out liquid. Stir potatoes into egg mixture.

3. Drop potato mixture by generous ⅓ cups, about 2 inches apart, onto prepared cookie sheet to make 12 mounds. Press each mound slightly to flatten into a 3-inch round.

4. Bake latkes 15 minutes. With wide metal spatula, turn latkes over and bake 15 minutes longer or until browned and crisp on both sides. Serve with applesauce if you like.

EACH SERVING (1 LATKE): ABOUT 65 CALORIES, 2 G PROTEIN, 15 G CARBOHYDRATE, 0 G TOTAL FAT (0 G SATURATED), 0 MG CHOLESTEROL, 160 MG SODIUM, 1 G FIBER

Traditional latkes
SINGLE SERVING: 150 CALORIES
Healthy Makeover Light Latkes
SINGLE SERVING: 65 CALORIES

You Save
85
CALORIES

Prevent holiday-season gain with these cold-weather calorie burners, from snowy chores and sports to festive indoor fun.

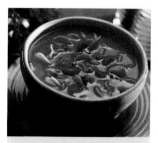

ACTIVITY	CALORIES Burned per Hour*
Shoveling your driveway	401
Ice skating	368
Downhill skiing	334
Building a snowman	301
Walking in a winter wonderland (3 mph)	234
Wrapping presents	134
Setting up the tree, then decorating it	100

*Calculations based on a 140-pound woman.

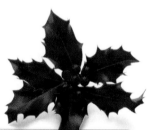

MAKE IT A HABIT
Start with Soup

Researchers have found that people who begin their meal with a broth-based soup can reduce their total calorie intake by a whopping 20 percent, compared with those who skip the soup. Why? Researchers speculate that even a low-calorie soup satisfies hunger because your brain perceives it as filling.

Drop

5 **DO IT NOW Step on the Scale** Get a close friend to watch you weigh yourself before **Thanksgiving** and **after New Year's.** When researchers weighed nineteen people before Thanksgiving and again in mid-January, participants' weights stayed the same—even though they consumed **36 percent more** calories, on average, over the holidays. Knowing they'd be accountable motivated volunteers to **shed the extra** pounds (either **through exercise** or **eating less** at other times), suggest the researchers.

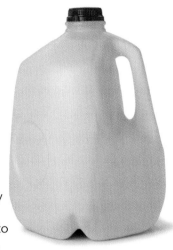

MAKE IT A HABIT
Be the Waiter or Waitress

Instead of accepting the humongous piles of food your great-aunt dishes out, offer to serve everyone at the table. That way, you choose how much ends up on your plate (and you get brownie points for being helpful).

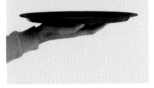

TOP 5 EASY HOLIDAY EXERCISES

The time you'd usually spend exercising now may well be spent shopping, wrapping, and baking instead. Try these quick, playful exercises—all will fit into a jam-packed schedule.

1. **MILK JUG SQUATS** When putting away groceries, grab a full, one-gallon container of milk or juice in each hand, then do six to eight squats (keep a straight back). It should feel like you're sitting down in an invisible chair, then standing up (if it helps, put a chair behind you, but don't sit down in it). Do at least two sets.

2. **GIFT WRAP RUNS** Wrap two gifts, then walk or run up and down your stairs three times or jog in place for two minutes. Repeat five times or until you're done packaging your presents.

3. **COOKIE PUSH-UPS** While you're waiting for the cookies to bake, do five push-ups (knees on the floor for beginners; plank position for advanced exercisers).

4. **SOUP CAN CURLS** While cooking, take an average-size soup can in each hand. Face your palms forward and "attach" your elbows to your waist. Then slowly raise one arm at a time to your chest and return it to the straight, hanging position. Do one set of ten repetitions with each arm.

5. **POST-FEAST WALK** After the holiday meal, plan to take a 45-minute walk with a friend or family member.

Light and Creamy Eggnog

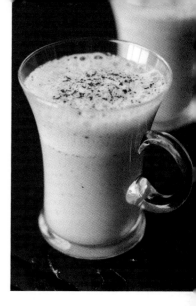

When it comes to holiday-time calories, perhaps nothing adds to your bottom line as much as this rich drink. But only a Scrooge would give up eggnog altogether, so check out our slimmed-down nog at one-fourth the saturated fat and calories. To skinny it down, we replaced whole milk with low-fat (and skipped the heavy cream) but kept the silky texture and decadent flavor by simmering the milk and sugar with cornstarch; we also used more egg whites and fewer yolks.

Active time 5 minutes
Total time 20 minutes
   plus chilling
Makes about 6½ cups or
13 servings

- 3 **large eggs**
- 3 **large egg whites**
- 5½ **cups low-fat (1%) milk**
- ½ **cup sugar**
- 2 **tablespoons cornstarch**
- ¼ **teaspoon salt**
- 2 **tablespoons vanilla extract**
- ½ **teaspoon grated nutmeg, plus additional for sprinkling**
- ⅓ **cup dark Jamaican rum (optional)**

1. In bowl, with whisk, beat eggs and egg whites until blended; set aside. In heavy 4-quart saucepan, with heat-safe spatula, mix 4 cups milk with sugar, cornstarch, and salt. Cook on medium-high until mixture boils and thickens slightly, stirring constantly. Boil 1 minute. Remove saucepan from heat.

2. Gradually whisk ½ cup simmering milk mixture into eggs; pour egg mixture back into milk in saucepan, whisking constantly, to make custard.

3. Pour custard into large bowl; stir in vanilla, nutmeg, rum (if using) and remaining 1½ cups milk. Cover and refrigerate until well chilled, at least 6 hours or up to 2 days. Sprinkle eggnog with nutmeg to serve.

EACH ½-CUP SERVING: ABOUT 105 CALORIES, 6 G PROTEIN, 14 G CARBOHYDRATE, 2 G TOTAL FAT (1 G SATURATED), 53 MG CHOLESTEROL, 125 MG SODIUM, 0 G FIBER

Classic eggnog
SINGLE SERVING: 440 CALORIES
Healthy Makeover
Light and Creamy Eggnog
SINGLE SERVING: 105 CALORIES

You Save
335
CALORIES

HEALTHY RECIPE MAKEOVER
Hot Cocoa Mix

On a wintry day, hot chocolate is the ultimate comfort-in-a-cup, whether you're still a kid or just a kid at heart. We make it Drop 5 friendly.

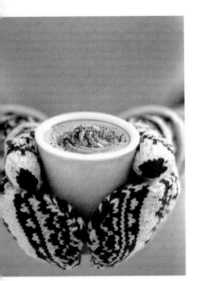

In food processor, with knife blade attached, blend 1¼ cups unsweetened cocoa, 1¼ cups sugar, 6 ounces coarsely chopped semisweet chocolate, and ¼ teaspoon salt until almost smooth. Store in tightly sealed container at room temperature up to 6 months.

To make For each serving, in a microwave-safe mug, mix 3 tablespoons mix with 1 cup nonfat milk. Microwave on High 1½ to 2 minutes or until blended and hot, stirring once. **115 CALORIES**

Mocha Variation Prepare Hot Cocoa Mix recipe, adding ⅓ **cup instant coffee powder or granules** before blending in processor.

Mexican Spice Variation Prepare Hot Cocoa Mix recipe, adding **2 teaspoons ground cinnamon** and ¼ **teaspoon ground red pepper (cayenne)** before blending in processor.

Vanilla Variation Prepare Hot Cocoa Mix recipe, adding ½ **vanilla bean (pod and seeds)** before blending in processor.

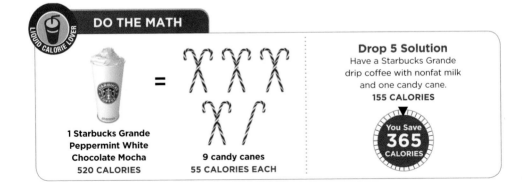

DO THE MATH

1 Starbucks Grande Peppermint White Chocolate Mocha
520 CALORIES

=

9 candy canes
55 CALORIES EACH

Drop 5 Solution
Have a Starbucks Grande drip coffee with nonfat milk and one candy cane.
155 CALORIES

You Save **365** CALORIES

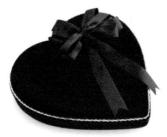

Valentine's Day Quick Quiz

Every Valentine's Day, your husband or partner buys you a big box of fancy chocolates. This year, you're trying to Drop 5. What do you do?

1. Accept the gift, but make a point of sharing it with coworkers or friends.

2. Tell him in advance that you'd rather he give you flowers.

3. Eat the chocolates (even if it's just one a day), fitting them into your Daily Calorie Targets (see page 212).

CORRECT ANSWER If you're committed to losing weight, tell your spouse or significant other before the holiday to skip the candy. First, let him know how much you appreciate his thoughtfulness. Then say, "Unfortunately, I love the chocolates so much that I'm afraid I'll eat them all, which would totally undo my efforts!" Suggest that something more diet friendly—say, flowers—would be better. Don't skirt the issue by accepting his gift and passing it on; you might hurt his feelings.

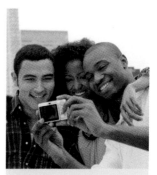

MAKE IT A HABIT
Keep Your Hands Occupied

Carry a clutch bag in one hand and a glass of sparkling water or a camera in the other, and you'll limit your chances of unconsciously snacking on party fare. Depending on the event, you can even designate yourself as an informal photographer for the occasion so that you stay busy and mingle with the other guests.

CRAVING 911

Craving
Cherry cordial candies

Try This
Chocolate-Dipped Strawberries

Swirl the bottom halves of three whole medium strawberries in melted chocolate (use half a semisweet chocolate square).

3 cherry cordial candies
165 CALORIES
3 Chocolate-Dipped Strawberries
75 CALORIES

You Save
90
CALORIES

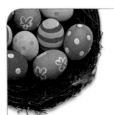

A Hard-Boiled (Easter) Egg

Crack open one of the kids' beautifully decorated hard-boiled eggs from the fridge, and enjoy it seasoned with salt and pepper (80 calories). Or make a deviled-egg with 1 tablespoon light mayonnaise, a pinch of paprika, and salt and pepper to taste; eat just half for 60 calories, or the whole deviled egg for 120.

MINDLESS MUNCHER | EASTER SWEETS CHEAT SHEET

A few jelly beans here, a Cadbury Creme Egg there—Easter basket calories can add up fast! Here, the skinny on calorie counts.

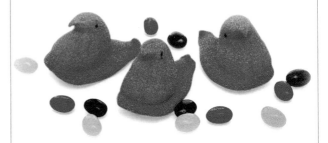

TREAT	CALORIES
1 Peeps Marshmallow Chick	28
10 small jelly beans	41
1 chocolate-covered marshmallow	42
12 Whoppers Mini Robin Eggs	96
1 Cadbury Creme Egg	170
1½-ounce solid chocolate bunny	230

JUNK FOOD JUNKIE | CRAVING 911

Craving	Try This
Cadbury Creme Egg	8 Whoppers Mini Robin Eggs

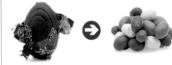

Tame your sweet tooth with 8 Whoppers Mini Robin Eggs. A crunchy malted milk ball interior coated by a very thin chocolate candy shell make these pretty speckled treats satisfying to munch.

Cadbury Creme Egg
170 CALORIES
8 Whoppers Mini Robin Eggs
64 CALORIES

You Save
106
CALORIES

Lighter Brownies

The rich texture and chocolate goodness of these bake-sale favorites speak of decadence, but compare each square's 95 calories and 3 grams of fat to a regular brownie's 206 calories and 11 grams of fat, and you'll feel virtuous (and satisfied). Our cheats? Swapping nonfat cocoa powder for chocolate and cholesterol-free spread for not-so-heart-healthy butter.

Brownies
SINGLE SERVING: 206 CALORIES
Healthy Makeover Lighter Brownies
SINGLE SERVING: 95 CALORIES

You Save
111
CALORIES

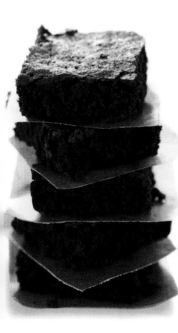

Active time 15 minutes
Total time 35 minutes
Makes 16 brownies

  Canola-oil nonstick cooking spray
1 **teaspoon instant coffee powder or granules**
2 **teaspoons vanilla extract**
½ **cup all-purpose flour**
½ **cup unsweetened cocoa**
¼ **teaspoon baking powder**
1¼ **teaspoons salt**
1 **cup sugar**
¼ **cup trans-fat free vegetable oil spread (60% to 70% oil)**
3 **large egg whites**

1. Preheat oven to 350°F. Grease 8-inch square metal baking pan with nonstick canola-oil cooking spray. In cup, dissolve coffee in vanilla extract.

2. On waxed paper, combine flour, cocoa, baking powder, and salt. In medium bowl, whisk sugar, vegetable oil spread, egg whites, and coffee mixture until well mixed; then blend in flour mixture. Spread in prepared pan.

3. Bake 22 to 24 minutes or until toothpick inserted in brownies 2 inches from edge comes out almost clean. Cool in pan on wire rack, about 2 hours.

4. When cool, cut brownies into 4 strips, then cut each strip crosswise into 4 squares. If brownies are difficult to cut, dip knife in hot water, wipe dry, and cut. Repeat dipping and drying as necessary.

EACH BROWNIE: ABOUT 95 CALORIES, 2 G PROTEIN, 17 G CARBOHYDRATE, 3 G TOTAL FAT (1 G SATURATED), 0 MG CHOLESTEROL, 75 MG SODIUM, 1 G FIBER

WARM WEATHER
gatherings

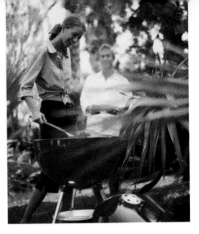

While winter holidays are notoriously dangerous for diets, summer celebrations, including Memorial Day, July Fourth, and Labor Day, as well as neighborhood barbecues, can also be calorie minefields.

TOP 5 TIPS FOR GUILT-FREE GRILLING

Grill parties don't have to spell trouble for your waistline. These tips can help you eat right but still savor the flavors.

1. **GO SKIN-FREE AND LOW-FAT** Grill skinless chicken, seafood, and lean cuts of beef, pork, or lamb, not high-fat hot dogs, hamburgers, and sausages.

2. **ADD CALORIE-FREE FLAVOR** Use flavored wood chips (like mesquite or apple wood) with coals to give food a nice smoky accent.

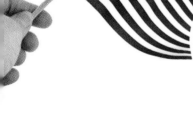

3. **PRETREAT THE MEAT** For tender, delicious chicken, marinate it in plain low-fat yogurt and mint; soak steak in soy sauce with fresh garlic. Try a "dry rub": Mix spices and herbs and rub on meat, poultry, or fish before grilling. Or brush on broth or nonfat salad dressing during grilling to keep fish and fresh vegetables moist.

4. **EAT YOUR VEGGIES** Load up on grilled corn on the cob, eggplant, summer squash, mushrooms, peppers, and other fresh vegetables.

5. **DON'T FORGET DESSERT** Grill cinnamon-dusted peach halves or pineapple wedges sprinkled with powdered ginger.

A BETTER BBQ

Having a calorie-conscious cookout starts in the grocery store and continues with your recipes. Here are easy ways to save big by choosing right.

Instead of traditional potato salad... → **...try Healthy Makeover Potato Salad**

DIET MADNESS	DIET MAKEOVER	YOU SAVE
Utz Sour Cream & Onion Dip **60 CALORIES PER** **2 TABLESPOONS**	Sour Cream and Onion Party Dip **45 CALORIES PER 2 TABLESPOONS** See recipe on page 242	**15** CALORIES
Traditional potato salad **215 CALORIES** **PER ⅔ CUP**	Healthy Makeover Potato Salad **150 CALORIES** **PER ⅔ CUP** See recipe on page 236	**65** CALORIES
Beef hot dog **185 CALORIES** **PER HOT DOG**	Hebrew National 97% Fat Free Beef Franks **45 CALORIES PER HOT DOG**	**140** CALORIES
Fried chicken breast with skin **364 CALORIES PER** **5-OUNCE BREAST**	Grilled chicken breast without skin **189 CALORIES PER** **4-OUNCE BREAST**	**175** CALORIES
Beef burger on a sesame-seed bun **485 CALORIES**	Veggie burger on a sesame-seed bun **250 CALORIES**	**235** CALORIES
Classic banana pudding **533 CALORIES** **PER ¼ CUP**	Better Banana Pudding **290 CALORIES PER ¼ CUP** See recipe on page 237	**243** CALORIES

HEALTHY RECIPE MAKEOVER
Potato Salad

This slimmed-down barbecue and picnic favorite saves a tidy sum of calories and fat over the traditional, mayo-loaded side dish—without sacrificing any of the flavor.

Active time 25 minutes
Total time 35 minutes
plus chilling
Makes 6 cups or 10 side-dish servings

- 3 **pounds Yukon Gold potatoes, peeled and cut into 1-inch chunks**
- 1¼ **teaspoons salt**
- ¾ **cup buttermilk**
- ¼ **cup light mayonnaise**
- 2 **tablespoons snipped fresh dill**
- 2 **tablespoons cider vinegar**
- 1 **tablespoon Dijon mustard**
- 2 **green onions, thinly sliced**
- ¼ **teaspoon coarsely ground black pepper**

1. In 4-quart saucepan, combine potatoes, 1 teaspoon salt, and enough *water* to cover; heat to boiling on high. Reduce heat to medium-low; cover and simmer 10 minutes or until potatoes are just fork-tender.

2. Meanwhile, in large bowl, whisk buttermilk with mayonnaise, dill, vinegar, mustard, green onions, remaining ¼ teaspoon salt, and pepper.

3. Drain potatoes well. Toss hot potatoes with buttermilk mixture until coated. (Mixture will look very loose before chilling.) Cover and refrigerate potato salad at least 2 hours (or overnight), stirring gently after 1 hour, to blend flavors.

EACH ⅔-CUP SERVING: ABOUT 150 CALORIES, 3 G PROTEIN, 29 G CARBOHYDRATE, 2 G TOTAL FAT (0.5 G SATURATED), 3 MG CHOLESTEROL, 200 MG SODIUM, 2 G FIBER

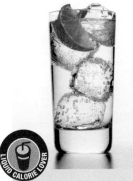

LIQUID CALORIE LOVER

MAKE IT A HABIT
Alternate Drinks

Drinking water or seltzer—both zero calories—between alcoholic drinks is a good way to slow your alcohol consumption and keep your weight loss on track.

Classic potato salad
SINGLE SERVING: 215 CALORIES
Healthy Makeover Potato Salad
SINGLE SERVING: 150 CALORIES

You Save
65
CALORIES

Better Banana Pudding

That innocent-looking banana pudding you grew up with is, alas, packed with calories. But here's a sweet reprieve: By halving the whipped cream and sugar, replacing four egg yolks with two whole eggs, and swapping in low-fat milk for whole, you save a lot of calories and 19 grams of fat per serving. Go ahead, have a dollop.

Classic banana pudding
SINGLE SERVING: 533 CALORIES
Healthy Makeover
Better Banana Pudding
SINGLE SERVING: 290 CALORIES

You Save
243
CALORIES

Total time 25 minutes
plus chilling
Makes 6 cups or 8 servings

- ⅓ cup plus 1 tablespoon **sugar**
- ¼ cup **cornstarch**
  Pinch salt
- 3 cups **low-fat (1%) milk**
- 2 **large eggs, lightly beaten**
- 1 teaspoon **vanilla extract**
- 40 **reduced-fat vanilla wafers (about half of one 11-ounce box)**
- 3 **ripe medium bananas, thinly sliced**
- ½ cup **heavy or whipping cream**

1. In 4-quart saucepan, combine ⅓ cup sugar with cornstarch and salt. Whisk in milk; heat to boiling on medium, stirring frequently. Gradually add eggs in thin, steady stream, beating vigorously with whisk to prevent curdling. Cook 1 minute, stirring. Remove saucepan from heat; stir vanilla into pudding.

2. In shallow 1½- to 2-quart casserole or serving dish, place 20 vanilla wafers; top with 1¼ cups pudding, spreading evenly, and half of banana slices. Repeat layering once, reserving 2 wafers for garnish. Top with remaining pudding, making sure to coat banana slices to prevent discoloration. Cover and refrigerate at least 8 hours or overnight.

3. When ready to serve, in medium bowl, with mixer on medium speed, beat cream and remaining 1 tablespoon sugar until stiff peaks form. Spread whipped cream over top of pudding. Coarsely crush reserved wafers and sprinkle over whipped cream.

EACH ¾-CUP SERVING: ABOUT 290 CALORIES, 7 G PROTEIN, 45 G CARBOHYDRATE, 10 G TOTAL FAT (5 G SATURATED), 77 MG CHOLESTEROL, 180 MG SODIUM, 1 G FIBER

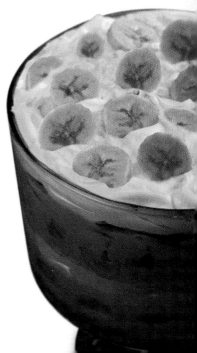

CELEBRATE OTHER
good times

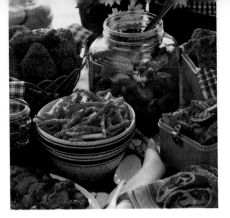

Whether it's a
birthday bash,
neighborhood shindig,
wedding reception,
Super Bowl party,
office get-together,
or any other event,
here's how to enjoy
the festivities with
your weight-loss
goal in mind.

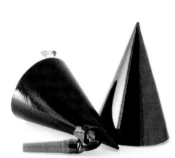

TOP 5 WAYS TO PARTY-PROOF YOUR DIET

1. **DON'T ARRIVE RAVENOUS** Before leaving the house, eat a little filling lean protein such as yogurt, cottage cheese, turkey, chicken, salmon, or water-packed tuna. This way, you'll have more resistance when you face tempting caloric fare.

2. **PRACTICE PORTION CONTROL** You can eat what you love, just not a lot of it. You'll feel more satisfied indulging in a small portion of three-cheese lasagna, say, than eating just veggies.

3. **PICK YOUR PLEASURES** Scan the food offerings and choose the three to five dishes that are the most appealing. Fill your plate with small tastes of these things, skip the other items on the buffet (or fill the rest of your plate with veggies or greens), and don't go back for more.

4. **CHECK YOUR HUNGER** Often, the desire to eat is not about hunger but rather how delicious the food tastes. If you're satisfied, don't automatically reach for that second hot dog or another slice of cake.

5. **TAKE A SEAT** When you're standing and chatting while eating, it's difficult to keep tabs on how much you're consuming. If possible, sit down at a table (preferably far away from the buffet), savor your food, and be mindful of what you are eating.

Have Your Cake and Drop 5 Too

Birthdays, weddings, showers, and lots of other celebratory occasions go hand-in-hand with calorie-rich cake. But no food is so high in fat or sugar that eating it *on occasion* is going to ruin your Drop 5 efforts.

And cake, just like doughnuts, pie, candy, and other weight-loss saboteurs, can be part of your diet as long as you make it fit within your daily Drop 5 calorie budget. This means eating less before or after consuming the cake, having just a small slice or a few bites, or upping your activity to burn off the extra calories.

For portion control, try bringing or serving cupcakes instead of a traditional cake, or if you're baking, try making a low-calorie confection like our Angel Food Cake (recipe on page 241).

MYTH BUSTER

Fiction It's best to starve yourself before an event. **Fact** This plan will backfire because you'll use the "I haven't eaten all day" excuse to stuff yourself when you arrive. Instead, save calories for a party by cutting back slightly at each meal for several days beforehand. Then, make the best use of your calorie allotment. For extra weight-loss insurance, increase your activity level a few days before and after a big event.

Nibble on This

Need some motivation to stop at just one or two hors d'oeuvres? Take a look at how fast a few bites can add up.

6 pigs in a blanket = **300 CALORIES**

6 bacon-wrapped dates = **450 CALORIES**

6 coconut shrimp = **630 CALORIES**

6 Chinese dumplings = **780 CALORIES**

6 curried meatballs = **1,200 CALORIES**

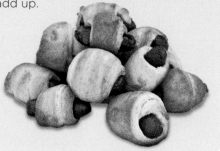

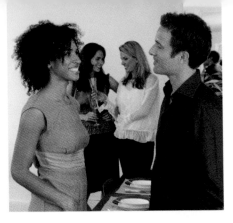

It's Not Just About the Food

Here are some more strategies on how to avoid the temptations of high-calorie bounty.

- Wear a form-fitting outfit, with a belt if possible. The snug fit will remind you not to stuff yourself to discomfort.

- Make socializing, rather than food, the focus of the event. Decide ahead of time that you will learn something new about someone you don't know well at the party.

- Put a special piece of jewelry on your hand or arm that you can see before the food goes onto your plate or into your mouth—a sparkly bangle or big ring, for example—as a visible reminder to yourself to eat in moderation.

- Practice saying "no, thank you," or stall with "not just yet." It's okay to turn down a rich dessert or tell an eager host you don't want seconds.

CRAVING 911

JUNK FOOD JUNKIE

Craving
Apple pie

Try This
Cinnamon Apple Delight

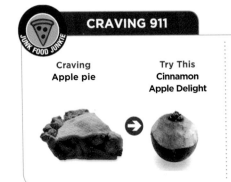

Core a cooking apple and peel one-third of the way down. Sprinkle the top with cinnamon, nutmeg, and 1 teaspoon brown sugar. Cook in the microwave, covered, on Medium-High (70% power) for 2 to 3 minutes, or until tender.

Apple pie
411 CALORIES
Cinnamon Apple Delight
115 CALORIES

You Save
295
CALORIES

Angel Food Cake

Beloved for its clean flavor and light texture, angel food cake has an added attraction—it's low in fat.

Active time 30 minutes
Total time 1 hour 5 minutes
Makes 16 servings

- 1 **cup cake flour (not self-rising)**
- ½ **cup confectioners' sugar**
- 1⅔ **cups egg whites (from 12 to 14 large eggs)**
- 1½ **teaspoons cream of tartar**
- ½ **teaspoon salt**
- 1¼ **cups granulated sugar**
- 2 **teaspoons vanilla extract**
- ½ **teaspoon almond extract**

1. Preheat oven to 375°F. Sift flour and confectioners' sugar through sieve set over small bowl.

2. In large bowl, with mixer at medium speed, beat egg whites, cream of tartar, and salt until foamy. Increase speed to medium-high; beat until soft peaks form when beaters are lifted. Sprinkle in granulated sugar, 2 tablespoons at a time, beating until sugar has dissolved and egg whites stand in stiff, glossy peaks when beaters are lifted. Beat in vanilla and almond extracts.

3. Transfer egg-white mixture to larger bowl. Sift flour mixture, one-third at a time, over beaten egg whites; fold in with rubber spatula just until flour mixture is no longer visible. Do not overmix.

4. Scrape batter into ungreased 9- to 10-inch tube pan; spread evenly. Bake until cake springs back when lightly pressed, 35 to 40 minutes. Invert pan with cake still inside onto large metal funnel or bottle; cool cake completely in pan. Run thin knife around cake to loosen from side and center tube of pan. Remove from pan and place on cake plate.

EACH SERVING: ABOUT 115 CALORIES, 3 G PROTEIN, 25 G CARBOHYDRATE, 0 G TOTAL FAT (0 G SATURATED), 0 MG CHOLESTEROL, 114 MG SODIUM, 0 G FIBER

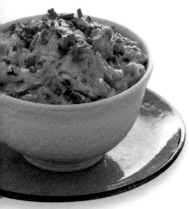

HEALTHY RECIPE MAKEOVER
Sour Cream and Onion Party Dip

You'll flip for this sour cream and onion dip. Store-bought tubs have more calories and fat—and they don't taste nearly as good as ours.

Active time 10 minutes
Total time 35 minutes
Makes 2 cups

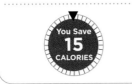

Classic sour cream and onion dip (such as Utz brand)
SINGLE SERVING: 60 CALORIES
Healthy Makeover Sour Cream and Onion Party Dip
SINGLE SERVING: 45 CALORIES

You Save
15
CALORIES

- 1½ **cups plain nonfat yogurt**
- 2 **tablespoons extra-virgin olive oil**
- 2 **medium yellow onions (6 to 8 ounces each), finely chopped**
- ¼ **teaspoon sugar**
- ¼ **teaspoon salt**
- ⅛ **teaspoon ground black pepper**
- ⅓ **cup reduced-fat sour cream**
  Snipped chives, for garnish
  Fresh veggie crudités, for serving

1. Line medium sieve set over deep bowl with basket-style coffee filter or paper towel. Spoon yogurt into filter; cover and refrigerate 25 minutes. Discard liquid in bowl.

2. Meanwhile, in 12-inch skillet, heat oil on medium until hot. Add onions, sugar, salt, and pepper. Cook 15 to 17 minutes or until dark golden brown, stirring onions occasionally.

3. Line plate with double thickness of paper towels. With slotted spoon, transfer onions to plate to drain further and cool. (Onions will crisp slightly as they cool, and a few pieces may stick to paper towel.)

4. In medium bowl, combine sour cream, strained yogurt, and onions. Stir well. Cover, and refrigerate at least 1 hour or up to 3 days. (Dip is best when refrigerated for a day; flavors develop more fully.) Garnish with chives and serve with fresh veggie crudités.

EACH 2-TABLESPOON SERVING: ABOUT 45 CALORIES, 2 G PROTEIN, 4 G CARBOHYDRATE, 2 G TOTAL FAT (1 G SATURATED), 2 MG CHOLESTEROL, 55 MG SODIUM, 1 G FIBER

PARTY CHEAT SHEET

Review these calorie counts before you hit the hazards of the cocktail party.

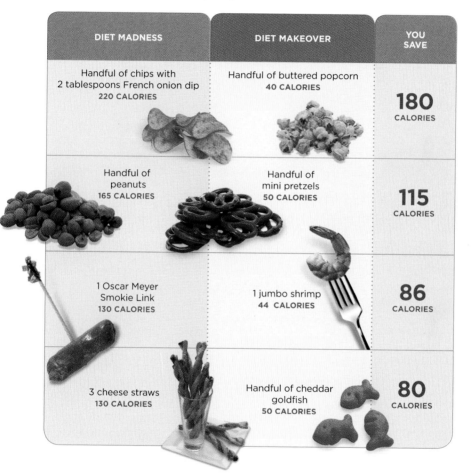

DIET MADNESS	DIET MAKEOVER	YOU SAVE
Handful of chips with 2 tablespoons French onion dip **220 CALORIES**	Handful of buttered popcorn **40 CALORIES**	**180** CALORIES
Handful of peanuts **165 CALORIES**	Handful of mini pretzels **50 CALORIES**	**115** CALORIES
1 Oscar Meyer Smokie Link **130 CALORIES**	1 jumbo shrimp **44 CALORIES**	**86** CALORIES
3 cheese straws **130 CALORIES**	Handful of cheddar goldfish **50 CALORIES**	**80** CALORIES

Drop

5 **DO IT NOW Chew Gum While You Tidy the Kitchen** During the post-feast kitchen cleanup, chomp on a piece of **sugarless gum** to keep you from **snacking** on leftovers. You can add a few hundred calories just by grazing on those **last few bites**.

good times

DRINK AT YOUR OWN RISK

Keep tabs on alcoholic beverages. Often, they're loaded with calories—especially the fancy concoctions—but don't have the benefit of filling you up. Even worse, alcohol lowers your inhibitions,

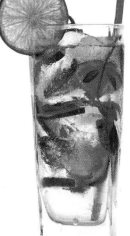

Instead of a Mojito at 220 calories...

BEVERAGE	CALORIES
Alcohol-free wine (5 ounces)	20–30
Beer (12 ounces)	150–200
Bloody Mary (5 ounces)	120
Champagne (4 ounces)	88
Tom Collins (8 ounces)	120
Coffee liqueur (3 ounces)	350
Cosmopolitan (4 ounces)	200
Godiva chocolate liqueur (3 ounces)	310
Gin and tonic (7 ounces)	200
Green apple martini (3 ounces)	150
Hot buttered rum (8 ounces)	300
Hot chocolate with peppermint schnapps (8 ounces)	380
Light beer (12 ounces)	100–145
Long Island iced tea (8 ounces)	780
Mai tai (4½ ounces)	350
Manhattan (2½ ounces)	130

making it more likely you'll go back for seconds (or thirds). That's why we suggest a 150-calorie cutoff, or about one drink for women. To see how quickly the calories from alcohol add up, consult the chart below. (See also "Happy House Alert" on page 132.)

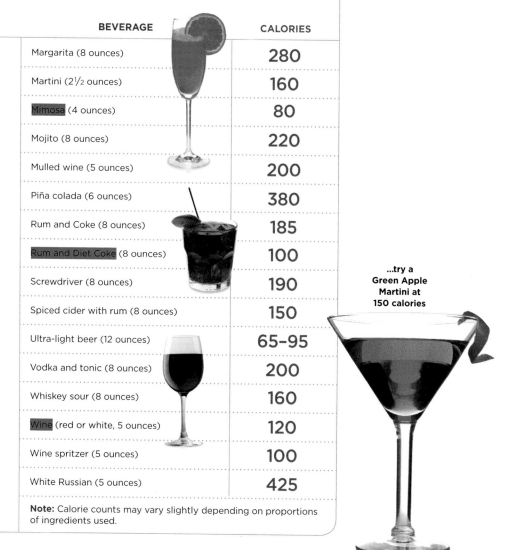

BEVERAGE	CALORIES
Margarita (8 ounces)	280
Martini (2½ ounces)	160
Mimosa (4 ounces)	80
Mojito (8 ounces)	220
Mulled wine (5 ounces)	200
Piña colada (6 ounces)	380
Rum and Coke (8 ounces)	185
Rum and Diet Coke (8 ounces)	100
Screwdriver (8 ounces)	190
Spiced cider with rum (8 ounces)	150
Ultra-light beer (12 ounces)	65–95
Vodka and tonic (8 ounces)	200
Whiskey sour (8 ounces)	160
Wine (red or white, 5 ounces)	120
Wine spritzer (5 ounces)	100
White Russian (5 ounces)	425

Note: Calorie counts may vary slightly depending on proportions of ingredients used.

...try a **Green Apple Martini** at **150 calories**

DROP 5 CALCULATOR WORKSHEETS

OUR **WORKSHEETS MAKE IT EASY** to keep track of your daily and weekly calorie cutting so you can achieve your weight-loss goal.

Just insert your chosen strategies and the calorie savings. Then multiply that amount by the repetitions per week to get your total drop in calories. Tally up the entries in the Total Drop in Calories column, and you'll get your total weekly drop in calories. Below the chart, we help you figure out how long it will take you to Drop 5 lbs.

We've provided an example here (and another one in the Introduction on page 19) for you to use as you fill in the worksheets that follow.

You might opt to try only one strategy or up to four, or even more. Feel free to change strategies as you discover the diet and exercise routines that work best for you. We've included enough work sheets for you to experiment with the many different ways you can Drop 5!

DROP 5 CALCULATOR WORKSHEET

DROP 5 STRATEGY	CALORIES SAVED OR BURNED	REPETITIONS PER WEEK	TOTAL DROP IN CALORIES
Swap regular soda for diet (page 36)	140	14 (twice a day)	1,960
Ride a stationary bike at a moderate pace for 30 minutes	234	2	468
Have a veggie burger instead of a fast-food deluxe hamburger	460	1	460

TOTAL CALORIES SAVED OR BURNED PER WEEK	2,896

HOW LONG WILL IT TAKE THIS DIETER TO DROP 5? Simply divide the drop in calories required to lose one pound **(3,500)** by the actual drop in calories in a week **(2,896)** and you'll get the time it will take to lose **1 pound:**

$$3{,}500 \div 2{,}896 = 1.2 \text{ WEEKS}$$

Multiply by 5 to find out how long it will take to lose **5 pounds:**

$$1.2 \times 5 = 6 \text{ WEEKS}$$

DROP 5 CALCULATOR WORKSHEET

DROP 5 STRATEGY	CALORIES SAVED OR BURNED	REPETITIONS PER WEEK	TOTAL DROP IN CALORIES
Strategy 1			
Strategy 2			
Strategy 3			
Strategy 4			

TOTAL CALORIES SAVED OR BURNED PER WEEK

HOW LONG WILL IT TAKE YOU TO DROP 5? Simply divide the drop in calories required to lose one pound **(3,500)** by the actual drop in calories in a week and you'll get the time it will take to lose **1 pound:**

$$3,500 \div \underline{\hspace{3cm}} = \underline{\hspace{2cm}} \text{ WEEKS}$$

Multiply by 5 to find out how long it will take to lose **5 pounds:**

$$\underline{\hspace{3cm}} \times 5 = \underline{\hspace{2cm}} \text{ WEEKS}$$

DROP 5 CALCULATOR WORKSHEET

DROP 5 STRATEGY	CALORIES SAVED OR BURNED	REPETITIONS PER WEEK	TOTAL DROP IN CALORIES
Strategy 1			
Strategy 2			
Strategy 3			
Strategy 4			

TOTAL CALORIES SAVED OR BURNED PER WEEK

HOW LONG WILL IT TAKE YOU TO DROP 5? Simply divide the drop in calories required to lose one pound **(3,500)** by the actual drop in calories in a week and you'll get the time it will take to lose **1 pound:**

$$3,500 \div \text{_____} = \text{_____} \text{ WEEKS}$$

Multiply by 5 to find out how long it will take to lose **5 pounds:**

$$\text{_____} \times 5 = \text{_____} \text{ WEEKS}$$

DROP 5 CALCULATOR WORKSHEET

DROP 5 STRATEGY	CALORIES SAVED OR BURNED	REPETITIONS PER WEEK	TOTAL DROP IN CALORIES
Strategy 1			
Strategy 2			
Strategy 3			
Strategy 4			

TOTAL CALORIES SAVED OR BURNED PER WEEK

HOW LONG WILL IT TAKE YOU TO DROP 5? Simply divide the drop in calories required to lose one pound **(3,500)** by the actual drop in calories in a week and you'll get the time it will take to lose **1 pound:**

3,500 ÷ _____ = _____ WEEKS

Multiply by 5 to find out how long it will take to lose **5 pounds:**

_____ x 5 = _____ WEEKS

DROP 5 CALCULATOR WORKSHEET

DROP 5 STRATEGY	CALORIES SAVED OR BURNED	REPETITIONS PER WEEK	TOTAL DROP IN CALORIES
Strategy 1			
Strategy 2			
Strategy 3			
Strategy 4			

TOTAL CALORIES SAVED OR BURNED PER WEEK

HOW LONG WILL IT TAKE YOU TO DROP 5? Simply divide the drop in calories required to lose one pound **(3,500)** by the actual drop in calories in a week and you'll get the time it will take to lose **1 pound:**

$$3,500 \div \text{_____} = \text{_____} \text{ WEEKS}$$

Multiply by 5 to find out how long it will take to lose **5 pounds:**

$$\text{_____} \times 5 = \text{_____} \text{ WEEKS}$$

DROP 5 CALCULATOR WORKSHEET

DROP 5 STRATEGY	CALORIES SAVED OR BURNED	REPETITIONS PER WEEK	TOTAL DROP IN CALORIES
Strategy 1			
Strategy 2			
Strategy 3			
Strategy 4			

TOTAL CALORIES SAVED OR BURNED PER WEEK

HOW LONG WILL IT TAKE YOU TO DROP 5? Simply divide the drop in calories required to lose one pound **(3,500)** by the actual drop in calories in a week and you'll get the time it will take to lose **1 pound:**

$$3{,}500 \div \underline{\hspace{2cm}} = \underline{\hspace{2cm}} \text{ WEEKS}$$

Multiply by 5 to find out how long it will take to lose **5 pounds:**

$$\underline{\hspace{2cm}} \times 5 = \underline{\hspace{2cm}} \text{ WEEKS}$$

DROP 5 CALCULATOR WORKSHEET

DROP 5 STRATEGY	CALORIES SAVED OR BURNED	REPETITIONS PER WEEK	TOTAL DROP IN CALORIES
Strategy 1			
Strategy 2			
Strategy 3			
Strategy 4			

TOTAL CALORIES SAVED OR BURNED PER WEEK

HOW LONG WILL IT TAKE YOU TO DROP 5? Simply divide the drop in calories required to lose one pound **(3,500)** by the actual drop in calories in a week and you'll get the time it will take to lose **1 pound:**

3,500 ÷ _____ = _____ WEEKS

Multiply by 5 to find out how long it will take to lose **5 pounds:**

_____ x 5 = _____ WEEKS

DROP 5 CALCULATOR WORKSHEET

DROP 5 STRATEGY	CALORIES SAVED OR BURNED	REPETITIONS PER WEEK	TOTAL DROP IN CALORIES
Strategy 1			
Strategy 2			
Strategy 3			
Strategy 4			

TOTAL CALORIES SAVED OR BURNED PER WEEK

HOW LONG WILL IT TAKE YOU TO DROP 5? Simply divide the drop in calories required to lose one pound **(3,500)** by the actual drop in calories in a week and you'll get the time it will take to lose **1 pound:**

$$3,500 \div \underline{\hspace{3cm}} = \underline{\hspace{2cm}} \text{ WEEKS}$$

Multiply by 5 to find out how long it will take to lose **5 pounds:**

$$\underline{\hspace{3cm}} \times 5 = \underline{\hspace{2cm}} \text{ WEEKS}$$

DROP 5 CALCULATOR WORKSHEET

DROP 5 STRATEGY	CALORIES SAVED OR BURNED	REPETITIONS PER WEEK	TOTAL DROP IN CALORIES
Strategy 1			
Strategy 2			
Strategy 3			
Strategy 4			

TOTAL CALORIES SAVED OR BURNED PER WEEK

HOW LONG WILL IT TAKE YOU TO DROP 5? Simply divide the drop in calories required to lose one pound **(3,500)** by the actual drop in calories in a week and you'll get the time it will take to lose **1 pound:**

$$3,500 \div \underline{\hspace{3cm}} = \underline{\hspace{2cm}} \text{ WEEKS}$$

Multiply by 5 to find out how long it will take to lose **5 pounds:**

$$\underline{\hspace{3cm}} \times 5 = \underline{\hspace{2cm}} \text{ WEEKS}$$

INDEX TO EATING BEHAVIORS... AND HOW TO CHANGE THEM

When you took the Diet Decoder Quiz (page 12), you discovered the principal eating behaviors or habits that may have undermined your weight-loss efforts in the past. Whether you are a Junk Food Junkie, a Liquid Calorie Lover, or some combination of the five different eating types described in the quiz, this index makes it easy to locate the recipes and strategies that will help you overcome your particular diet pitfalls.

NOTE: PAGE NUMBERS IN *ITALICS* INDICATE RECIPES.

EMOTIONAL EATERS use food for more than fuel—it also serves as a friend and a comfort.

about: calculating your score, 14; definition and icon, 15
basics of emotional eating, 71
Better Banana Pudding, *237*
Chocolate Chip Cookies, *70*
coping alternatives, 71
Craving 911, 64
Creamy Mushroom Cavatappi, *175*
keeping food diary, 64
Learn from the "Losers," 35
Light Latkes, *226*
Meat Loaf, *57*
Poached Pears with Fresh Ginger, *179*
Shepherd's Pie, *67*
Strawberry Ice Cream, *69*
stress management and, 71, 126, 216
sweet makeovers, 178
triggers, 71
types of hunger and, 100
Whole-Wheat Penne Genovese, *177*

Empty-Calorie Exercise Calculator, 199
Fast Food Exercise Calculator, 201
50-calorie sweet snacks, 52
food/exercise diary and, 217
Halloween, seasonal candy and, 214–215, 217
healthy frozen desserts, 106–107
ice cream swaps, 107
keeping treats out of sight, 112
Learn from the "Losers," 71
Lighter Brownies, *233*
McDonald's breakfast picks, 150
not eating enough produce, 94
party cheat sheet, 243
pastries and baked goods, 148, 150, 152, 239
pie types and calories per piece, 225
pizza choices, 60
Poached Pears with Fresh Ginger, *179*
Pumpkin Spice Ring, *224*
purging pantry, 34
quick-fix treats, 68
reducing sugar, 80
shopping online, 77
Sour Cream and Onion Party Dip, *242*
terrifying treats, 214
vending machine know-how, 120

JUNK FOOD JUNKIES fill up on nutrient-poor, empty-calorie foods.

about: calculating your score, 14; definition and icon, 15
Angel Food Cake, *241*
candy bars and calories, 214–215
chicken done right, 161
cookout makeover savings, 235
Craving 911s, 44, 93, 231, 232, 240
dieting on doughnuts, 148
eating dried plums (prunes), 129

LIQUID CALORIE LOVERS unwittingly load their diet with extra calories from drinks.

about: calculating your score, 14; definition and icon, 15
alcoholic beverage calories, 244–245
beverage exercise calculator, 200
buying whole fruits instead of juices, 34, 83
calorie-burning drinks, 83
calorie-reduction chart, 82
coffee break calories, 153

coffee drink makeover, 151, 230
drinking water/seltzer between alcoholic
    drinks, 236
happy hour tips, 132–133, 244–245
Hot Cocoa Mix, *230*
instantly cutting eating-out calories, 157
keeping/drinking water at your desk, 128
making café au lait, 42
mistaking thirst for hunger, 120
Light and Creamy Eggnog, 229
smoothie calories (by vendor), 154
Strawberry Mania, *155*
swaps/substitutions, 34–37, 54, 82
switching to 1 percent or nonfat milk, 103
veggie juice benefits, 64

Starbucks breakfast picks, 146
starving-before-event myth, 239
Subway sandwiches, 160
workplace snacks, 121

MINDLESS MUNCHERS are unconscious eaters and all-day grazers who eat out of habit or boredom, regardless of hunger.

about: calculating your score, 14; definition and
    icon, 15
appetizer calorie savings, 166, 239
buffet control and, 213
candy calorie savings, 127
carrying mint sprig during holidays, 220
checking your hunger, 238
chewing gum when cleaning kitchen, 243
curbing all-day nibbling, 122
Easter sweets cheat sheet, 232
eating when bored, 131
Guiltless Guacamole, *167*
hors d'oeuvres calories, 239
keeping your hands occupied, 231
Learn from the "Losers," 55, 95, 100, 152
100-calorie comparison, 53
not eating what you don't want, 117
party-proofing diet, 238
practicing portion control, 144–145
savoring meal memories, 119
snacking smarter, 81
Sour Cream and Onion Party Dip, *242*
stocking house with calorie-controlled
    snacks, 53
taking quick walks, 123
tracking wrappers, 214

MEAL SKIPPERS often wait too long between meals. As a result, they frequently end up making poor diet choices and caving in on cravings because they're so famished.

about: calculating your score, 14; definition and
    icon, 15
breakfast tips, 38, 114–115, 146–150
50-calorie healthy snacks, 52
friendly fast food, 147, 160
healthy convenience fruits and vegetables, 94
healthy convenience grain dishes, 85
healthy convenience seafood, 100
healthy convenience snacks, 81
healthy frozen heat-and-eat sandwiches, 105
healthy frozen meals and pizza, 105
100-calorie munchies, 54–55
party-proofing diet, 238
preprepped produce, 90
Quiznos sandwiches, 160
slow-cooking tips, 61

EAT MORE FIBER INDEX

Eating more fiber is an excellent Drop 5 strategy for everyone. Fiber fills you up without adding extra calories, which means eating meals built around fiber-rich food such as beans, fruit, veggies, and whole grains makes it a lot less likely you'll overeat. To help you find fiber-rich foods fast, here is a list of all meals, recipes, and snacks in the book that are an excellent source of fiber (they have 5 grams of fiber or more per serving), plus fiber-friendly tips.

NOTE: PAGE NUMBERS IN *ITALICS* INDICATE RECIPES.

Appetizer, Black Bean Dip meal, 50
Breakfast. *See also* Cereal
about: instant oatmeal options, 42
Berry Parfait, *114*
Black Bean and Salsa Omelet meal, *40*
French Toast meal, 43
Frittata, *38*
Fruit and Cheese, *114*
Garden Vegetable Omelet meal, *40*
Hot Cereal with Fruit, *38*
Red Pepper and Goat Cheese Omelet meal, *41*
Spinach, Cheese, and Bacon Omelet meal, *41*
Starbucks picks, 146
Sweet and Salty, *115*
Western-Style Omelet meal, *41*
Cereal
adding fruit to, 86
Cereal and Fruit, *114*
healthy options (by brand), 86
Hot Cereal with Fruit, *38*
instant oatmeal options, 42
Oatmeal with Apples and Pecans, *114*
Fiber, defined, 24
Frozen food, 105
Grains. *See also* Cereal
about: importance of, 56
Daily Calorie Targets and, 17
healthy convenience dishes (by brand), 85
shopping for, 84–87
truth about, 84
whole, 23, 84

Labels, reading, 24
Lunches, 116, 157, 160. *See also* Main dishes
Main dishes
about: healthy frozen meals, 105
Black-Eyed Pea Sauté meal, *51*
Chicken and Artichoke Pasta, *98*
Chicken Breasts Provençal meal, *63*
Chicken Breasts with Apple-Curry Sauce meal, *62*
Chicken Breasts with Black Bean Salsa meal, *63*
Chicken Breasts with Chinese Ginger Sauce meal, *63*
Chicken Breasts with Dijon Sauce meal, *62*
Confetti Pasta meal, *58*
Creamy Mushroom Cavatappi meal, *175*
Marinara Pasta meal, *59*
Meat Loaf meal, *57*
Mediterranean Couscous, *98*
Orange-Fennel Pasta meal, *58*
Pasta with Peas and Onion meal, *59*
Pasta with Tomatoes and Lemon meal, *59*
Pasta with Tuna Puttanesca, *79*
Shepherd's Pie meal, *67*
Shrimp Rice with Baby Peas, *92*
Snow Pea Stir-Fry, *92*
Spinach and Tortellini, *91*
Spinach and White Bean Pasta, *91*
Steak Fried Rice, *101*
Steak Pesto Pasta, *101*
Thai Steak Noodles, *101*
Turkey Fajitas meal, *171*
Whole-Wheat Penne Genovese, *177*

Salads
Chicken and Rice Salad, *45*
Chicken Pasta Salad with Chicken and Mixed Veggies, *92*
Dijon Bean and Veggie Salad, *45*
Garbanzo Bean Salad meal, 50
Greek Steak Salad, *101*
Honey Mustard Chicken Salad, *45*
Lime Tuna and Black Bean Salad, *45*
Salmon and Black Bean Tortilla Salad, *79*
Spinach Salad with Chicken, *91*
Sweet and Savory Salmon Salad, *45*
Tuna Salad, *48*
Tuscan Tuna Salad, *79*
Waldorf Salad, *98*
Sandwiches
about: 450-calorie sandwich, 46–47; frozen heat-and-eat option, 105
Caribbean Wrap, *98*
Greek Chicken Burgers meal, *173*
Open-Faced Chicken Quesadilla, *98*
Open-Faced Mexican Veggie Burrito, *92*
Spinach and Hummus Flatbread, *91*
Tuna English Muffins, *79*
Tuna Salad, *48*
Soups
about: healthy canned soup, 78
Black Bean Soup meal, *51*
Kidney Bean Chili meal, *51*
New England Clam Chowder, *66*
Vegetables, healthy convenience option, 94

GENERAL INDEX

NOTE: PAGE NUMBERS IN
ITALICS INDICATE RECIPES.

Alcohol, calories and, 132–133, 170, 244–245
All-or-nothing attitude, 213
Almost Bagel, *38*
Angel Food Cake, *241*
Appetizers
  eating out (by vendor), 166
  hors d'oeuvres calories, 239
  list of healthy recipes, 32. *See also specific recipes or main ingredients*
Apple-Curry Sauce, *62*
Asian food, 168–169
Attention on what you eat. *See* Conscious eating

Ballet, 203
Balsamic Berries, *68*
Bananas
  Bar Breakfast, *115*
  Better Banana Pudding, *237*
  PB and B, *115*
Bar Breakfast, *115*
Beans and legumes
  about: canned beans 5 easy ways, 50–51; hummus, 47, 52, 172; nutritional value of, 158; on salad bar, 158
  Black Bean and Salsa Omelet, *40*
  Black Bean Dip, *50*
  Black Bean Salsa, *63*
  Black Bean Soup, *51*
  Black-Eyed Pea Sauté, *51*
  Dijon Bean and Veggie Salad, *45*
  Garbanzo Bean Salad, *50*
  Guiltless Guacamole, *167*
  Kidney Bean Chili, *51*
  Lean Green Bean Casserole, *221*
  Lime Tuna and Black Bean Salad, *45*
  Open-Faced Mexican Veggie Burrito, *92*
  Pasta with Peas and Onion, *59*
  Salmon and Black Bean Tortilla Salad, *79*
  Snow Pea Stir-Fry, *92*

Spinach and White Bean Pasta, *91*
Beef. *See* Meat
Berries
  about: strawberries, 88
  Balsamic Berries, *68*
  Berry Parfait, *114*
  Blueberry Muffins, *39*
  Strawberry Ice Cream, *69*
  Strawberry Mania (smoothie), *155*
Better Banana Pudding, *237*
Beverages. *See* Drinks
Black beans. *See* Beans and legumes
Black-Eyed Pea Sauté, *51*
Book overview, 8–9
Boredom, eating and, 131
Breads. *See also* Sandwiches
  about: healthy crackers and (by brand), 87
  Almost Bagel, *38*
  Blueberry Muffins, *39*
  Sweet and Salty, *115*
Breakfast
  easy at-home, 114
  eating in, 38–43
  grab-and-go, 115
  list of healthy recipes, 32. *See also specific recipes or main ingredients*
  on-the-job, 115
  skipping, weight loss and, 115
  smoothies, *115*, 154, *155*
  three-day meal plan, 20–21
  work and, 114–115
Breakfast (eating out), 146–155
  best in bakery (by vendor), 152
  coffee break calories (by vendor), 153
  coffee drink makeover (by vendor), 151
  diner meals/calories (by vendor), 149
  doughnuts/calories (by vendor), 148
  Eating Out Calorie IQ, 140–141
  food court report (by vendor), 142

friendly fast food/calories (by vendor), 147
  McDonald's picks, 150
  ordering à la carte, 154
  pastries and baked goods, 148, 150, 152
  Starbucks picks, 146
Broccoli
  about, 89
  Broccoli-Cheddar Scramble, *92*
Brown bag lunches, 110–111, 116
Brussels sprouts, about, 89
Buffet behaviors, 164, 213

Café au Lait, *42*
Calorie-burning drinks, 83
Calories, 16–19. *See also specific foods*
  calculating, 19
  consumption comparison, 53
  creating deficit for weight loss, 10
  cutting drastically, 10
  Daily Calorie Targets, 16, 17, 30, 77, 113, 138, 212
  Drop 5 Calculator, 19
  easiest ways to burn 100, 204
  Eating Out Calorie IQ, 140–141
  Empty-Calorie Exercise Calculator, 199
  laughing and burning, 206
  optimizing, 22–23
  Out-to-Lunch Calorie IQ (by vendor), 118
  per pound of weight, 10
  reading labels, 24, 76
  standing vs. sitting and, 205
  trimming from home-cooked meals, 28–29
Candy. *See* Snacks
Canned and dry goods, shopping for, 78–80
Caribbean Wrap, *98*
Cereal
  fruit and, *38*, 86, *114*
  healthy options (by brand), 86
  instant oatmeal options, 42
Cheese. *See* Dairy

Chicken
    about: breasts 5 easy ways,
      62; fast-food best choices
      (by vendor), 161; in salads,
      159; shopping for meat,
      seafood and, 96–101; thighs,
      99; top 5 meal ideas for
      rotisserie, 98
    Breasts Provençal, *63*
    Breasts with Apple-Curry
      Sauce, *62*
    Breasts with Black Bean
      Salsa, *63*
    Breasts with Chinese Ginger
      Sauce, *63*
    Breasts with Dijon Sauce, *62*
    Caribbean Wrap, *98*
    Chicken and Artichoke
      Pasta, *98*
    Chicken and Rice Salad, *45*
    Greek Chicken Burgers, *173*
    Honey Mustard Chicken
      Salad, *45*
    Open-Faced Chicken
      Quesadilla, *98*
    Pasta Salad with Chicken and
      Mixed Veggies, *92*
    Red-Cooked Chicken with
      Assorted Vegetables, *61*
    Waldorf Salad, *98*
Chinese food, 168–169
Chinese Ginger Sauce, *63*
Chocolate
    Chocolate Chip Cookies, *70*
    Chocolate Figs, *68*
    Hot Cocoa Mix, *230*
    Lighter Brownies, *233*
Coffee
    Café au Lait, *42*
    Coffee Granita, *68*
    drink makeover
      (by vendor), 151
Coffee break calories (by
    vendor), 153
Condiment must-haves, 36
Confetti Pasta, *58*
Conscious eating, 31, 137, 139, 238
Craving 911
    apple pie, 240
    cherry cordial candies, 231
    Chinese fried rice, 164
    Easter candy, 233

French fries, 44
    pot pies, 64
    strawberry shortcake, 93
Cravings
    being at peace with, 213
    importance of controlling, 31
Creamy Mushroom
    Cavatappi, *175*
Crunchy Fruit Creation, *115*

Daily Calorie Targets, 16, 17, 30,
    77, 113, 138, 212
Dairy. *See also* Eggs
    calcium-rich diets, weight
      loss and, 103
    cheese in salads, 159
    healthy cheeses
      (by brand), 102
    healthy frozen desserts (by
      brand), 106–107
    healthy yogurt (by brand), 103
    low-fat, 23, 102, 103
    100-calorie snacks, 55
    shopping tips, 102–104
    switching to 1 percent or
      nonfat milk, 103
    trimming fat and calories,
      28–29
Desserts
    eating out (by vendor), 178
    healthy frozen (by brand),
      106–107
    ice cream swaps (by brand),
      106, 107
    list of healthy recipes, 33. *See*
      also specific recipes or main
      ingredients
    pie types and calories per
      piece, 225
    reducing sugar intake
      and, 80
Diary, food, 64, 217
Diet Decoder Quiz
    eating behaviors icons and
      descriptions, 15. *See also*
      Index to Eating Behaviors
    questions, 12–14
    tallying results, 14
Diets, 8
Diet Traps
    about: overview of, 11
    avoiding new foods, 76

buffets, 164
discounting little things, 126
eating when bored, 131
keeping treats visible, 112
mistaking thirst for
    hunger, 120
not counting alcohol
    calories, 170
not eating enough
    produce, 94
skimping on sleep, 124
waiting until January 1 to
    change habits, 220
Dijon Bean and Veggie Salad, *45*
Dijon Sauce, *62*
Dinner
    eating in, 56–67
    eating veggies/salad first, 56
    list of healthy recipes, 32–33.
      See also specific recipes or
      main ingredients
    three-day meal plan, 20–21
Dinner (eating out), 164–177
    appetizers (by vendor), 166
    Asian food, 168
    buffet behaviors, 164
    chain restaurant
      recommendations (by
      vendor), 176
    Eating Out Calorie IQ,
      140–141
    food court report (by
      vendor), 143
    Greek food, 172
    hall of shame pasta dishes
      (by vendor), 174
    Italian food, 174, 176
    menu key words and, 165
    Mexican food, 170
    steak cuts/calories, 165
Dogs, walking, 207
Do It Now
    eating in, 49, 53, 60
    eating out, 144–145, 157, 165
    fitness, 189, 190, 196, 206
    on the job, 113, 117, 125, 128,
      129, 130
    supermarket savvy, 80, 81, 86
    sweet celebrations, 214, 220,
      227, 243
Do the Math calculations, 106,
    119, 148, 217, 225, 230

Drinks
  alcoholic, calories, 132–133,
    170, 244–245
  Beverage Exercise Calculator
    (by vendor), 200
  calorie-burning, 83
  list of healthy recipes, 32
  mistaking thirst for hunger, 120
  shopping for snacks
    and, 81–83
  smoothies, *115*, 154, *155*
  swapping fruits for
    juices, 34, 83
  swaps/substitutions
    (by brand), 82
  veggie juice benefits, 64
Drop 5 Calculator, 19
Drop 5 Calculator Worksheets,
  246–255
Dry and canned goods, shopping
  for, 78–80

Easter sweets and eggs, 232
Eating behaviors. *See also* Index
  to Eating Behaviors
  descriptions and icons, 15
  Diet Decoder Quiz and, 12–14
Eating in
  about: overview of, 27
  breakfast, 38–43
  cleaning kitchen and, 28,
    34–37, 243
  controlling cravings, 31
  Daily Calorie Targets and, 30
  Do It Now, 49, 53, 60
  downsizing dishes, 30
  list of healthy recipes, 32–33.
    See also specific recipes or
    main ingredients
  lunch, 44–51
  Make It a Habit, 56, 64
  must-have foods, 35–37
  paying attention when, 31
  purging pantry and, 34
  snacks, 52–55
  substituting ingredients to
    trim fat and calories, 28–29
  sweets, 68–71
  top 5 how-tos, 28–31
Eating out. *See also* Breakfast
  (eating out); Dinner (eating
  out); Lunch (eating out)

about: overview of, 135
balancing choices, 138–139
calorie IQ, 140–141
consciously, 137
cutting calories when, 157
Daily Calorie Targets and, 138
damage control, 139
Do It Now, 144–145, 157, 165
Eating Out Calorie IQ. *See*
  also Eating out
Fast Food Exercise
  Calculator (by vendor), 201
food court report (by
  vendor), 142–143
Learn from the "Losers,"
  152, 162
learning about
  establishments, 136
managing hunger, 137
portion control guidelines,
  144–145
snacks, 142
top 5 how-tos, 136–139
Eating Out Calorie IQ, 140–141
Eggs
  about: cholesterol myth,
    104; for Easter, 232; hard-
    boiled, in salads, 159;
    nutritional value of, 104
  Black Bean and Salsa
    Omelet, *40*
  Broccoli-Cheddar
    Scramble, *92*
  Egg Rollup, *115*
  French Toast, *43*
  Frittata, *38*
  Garden Vegetable Omelet, *40*
  Light and Creamy
    Eggnog, *229*
  Red Pepper and Goat Cheese
    Omelet, *41*
  Spinach, Cheese, and Bacon
    Omelet, *41*
  Spinach Scramble, *91*
  Western-Style Omelet, *41*
Emotional Eaters. *See* Index to
  Eating Behaviors
Empty-Calorie Exercise
  Calculator, 199
Exercise. *See also* Fitness
  aerobic, 182, 203
  ballet, 203

Beverage Exercise Calculator
  (by vendor), 200
breaking up workouts,
  184–185
clothing affecting sweat
  levels and, 190
duration of, 207
easiest ways to burn 100
  calories, 204
Empty-Calorie Exercise
  Calculator, 199
family style, 183–184
Fast Food Exercise
  Calculator (by vendor), 201
fresh air and, 189
holiday-season activities,
  227, 228
holidays/sweet celebrations
  and, 211
in hotel room, 130
learning new skill, 184
low-sweat workouts, 202–203
measuring results, 190
music and, 206
pace of, 185, 188, 190
Pilates, 202
pleasure principle and, 183
pre-workout munchies, 198
scheduling/timing, 184–185,
  188, 196, 204, 205, 207
snacks and, 198–201
spot-reducing for weight loss
  and, 197
standing sit-up equivalent, 216
strength training, 192–197
stride and counting steps,
  190–191
Tai Chi, 203
team sports and, 206
25-minute at-work
  workout, 122
walking, 122, 186–191, 216
walking dogs and, 207
water workouts, 203
at work, 112, 122–123, 128, 130
yoga, 126, 203

Family participation, 75,
  183–184
Fast food. *See* Breakfast (eating
  out); Dinner (eating out);
  Eating out; Lunch (eating out)

Fats
  healthy, what to look for, 23
  omega-3s in fish, 99
  substituting ingredients to
    optimize, 28–29
Fiber. *See* Eat More Fiber Index;
  Grains
Fish and seafood
  about: eating more, 65;
    healthy convenience
    options (by brand), 100;
    omega-3s in, 99; shopping
    for meat, poultry and, 96–
    101; sushi mix up (by type),
    162; top meal ideas for
    canned fish, 79; trimming
    fat and calories, 28–29
  Lime Tuna and Black Bean
    Salad, 45
  New England Clam
    Chowder, 66
  Pasta with Tuna
    Puttanesca, 79
  Roasted Salmon with
    Squash, 65
  Salmon and Black Bean
    Tortilla Salad, 79
  Salmon Cakes, 79
  Sesame Shrimp and
    Asparagus Stir-Fry, 169
  Shrimp Rice with Baby
    Peas, 92
  Sweet and Savory Salmon
    Salad, 45
  Tuna English Muffins, 79
  Tuna Salad, 48
  Tuscan Tuna Salad, 79
Fitness. *See also* Exercise
  about: overview of, 181–182
  Do It Now, 189, 190, 196, 206
  e-mails inspiring, 128
  genes, metabolism, weight
    and, 182
  importance of, 25
  Learn from the "Losers," 55,
    123, 129, 191, 205, 207
  Make It a Habit, 187
  meditation, yoga and, 126, 203
  monitoring with PDA, 131
  Myth Busters, 197, 205, 207
  stress management and, 126
  team sports and, 206

top 5 tips, 183–185
traveling and, 130
Websites, 197
whittling your middle, 196
Food diary, 64, 217
Freezer must-haves, 37
Frittata, 38
Frozen food
  adding fresh produce to
    meals, 90
  desserts (by brand), 106–107
  healthy heat-and-eat
    sandwiches (by brand), 105
  healthy meals and pizzas (by
    brand), 105
  nutritional value of, 93
  shopping for (by brand),
    105–107
  top 5 vegetable meal ideas, 92
  at work, 116
Fruits. *See also specific fruits*
  about: adding to cereal,
    38, 86, 114; frozen, 93;
    healthiest, 88; not eating
    enough, 94; 100-calorie
    snacks, 54; prepped,
    90; in salads, 158. *See
    also* Salads; shopping for
    vegetables and, 88–95;
    swapping for juices, 34, 83
  Crunchy Fruit Creation, 115
  Fruit and Cheese, 114

Garbanzo beans. *See* Beans
  and legumes
Garden Vegetable Omelet, 40
Ginger Sauce, Chinese, 63
Grains. *See also* Cereal; Eat
  More Fiber Index; Pasta
  about: importance of, 56
  Daily Calorie Targets and, 17
  healthy convenience dishes
    (by brand), 85
  Mediterranean Couscous, 98
  rice stir-fry idea, 164
  shopping for, 84–87
  truth about, 84
  whole, 23, 84
Grapefruit, about, 88
Greek Chicken Burgers, 173
Greek food, 172–173
Greek Steak Salad, 101

Greens, about, 89, 158
Grilling, guilt-free tips, 234
Grocery shopping. *See* Shopping
  (supermarket savvy)
Guiltless Guacamole, 167

Halloween help, 215, 217
Holiday Herb-Roasted
  Potatoes, 218
Holidays. *See Sweet celebrations
  references*
Honey Mustard Chicken Salad, 45
Hot Cereal with Fruit, 38
Hot Cocoa Mix, 230
Hummus, 47, 52, 91, 116, 172
Hunger, managing, 137

Ice cream, 106–107
Ingredients. *See also specific
  main ingredients*
  buying. *See* Supermarket
    savvy
  must-have foods, 37–39
Italian food, 174–177

Junk Food Junkies. *See* Index to
  Eating Behaviors

Kidney beans. *See* Beans
  and legumes
Kitchen
  cleaning up, 28, 34–37, 243
  must-have foods, 35–37
Kiwifruit, about, 88

Labels, reading, 24, 76
Laughing, burning calories
  and, 206
Lean Green Bean Casserole, 221
Learn from the "Losers"
  eating-in tips, 37, 55, 71, 100
  eating-out tips, 152, 162
  fitness tips, 55, 123, 129, 191,
    205, 207
  on-the-job tips, 123, 129
  substitution tips, 152
  supermarket savvy, 35, 37,
    95, 100
Leftovers, 222
Light and Creamy Eggnog, 229
Lighter Brownies, 233
Light Latkes, 226

Liquid Calorie Lovers. *See* Index to Eating Behaviors
Lunch
eating in, 44–51
450-calorie sandwich, 46–47
list of recipes for, 32–33. *See also specific recipes or main ingredients*
Out-to-Lunch Calorie IQ (by vendor), 118
three-day meal plan, 20–21
at work, 116–121
Lunch (eating out), 156–163. *See also* Eating out
chicken done right (by vendor), 161
Eating Out Calorie IQ, 140–141
food court report (by vendor), 143
Quiznos choices, 160
sandwich do's, 156
slimming salads (by vendor), 163
sub shops and, 160
Subway choices, 160
sushi mix up (by type), 162
top salad bar choices, 158–159
winning meals (by vendor), 157

Main-dish recipe list, 32–33
Make It a Habit
eating in, 56, 64
fitness, 187
on the job, 117, 122, 128, 131
supermarket savvy, 83, 90, 103
sweet celebrations, 217, 222, 227, 228, 231, 236, 240
Marinara Pasta, *59*
meal Skippers. *See* Index to Eating Behaviors
Meat
about: calorie-conscious cuts, 97; healthy convenience options (by brand), 96; pork, 99; shopping for poultry, seafood and, 96–101; steak cuts/calories, 165; surprising good-for-your-waist picks, 99; tenderloin

steaks, 99; top 5 meal ideas for flank steak, 101; trimming fat and calories, 28–29
Greek Steak Salad, *101*
Meat Loaf, *57*
Shepherd's Pie, *67*
Steak Fajita Wraps, *101*
Steak Fried Rice, *101*
Steak Pesto Pasta, *101*
Thai Steak Noodles, *101*
Mediterranean Couscous, *98*
Mediterranean flavors, 172
Menus, three-day meal plan, 20–21
Metric equivalent charts, 268–269
Mexican food, 170–171
Mindful eating. *See* Conscious eating
Mindless Munchers. *See* Index to Eating Behaviors
Mint aroma, benefits of, 220
Mushrooms, in Creamy Mushroom Cavatappi, *175*
Music, fitness and, 206
Must-have foods, 37–39
Myth Busters
breakfast pastries being out, 148
carbs spelling trouble, 49
clothing increasing sweat in workouts, 190
egg cholesterol being bad, 104
fat-burning exercise requiring 20+ minutes, 207
food combinations helping slimming, 119
frozen fruit/vegetables being less nutritious, 93
genes determining metabolism and weight, 182
low-fat dairy being less nutritious, 102
morning being best exercise time, 205
skipping breakfast helping weight loss, 115
spot-reducing for weight loss, 197

New England Clam Chowder, *66*
Nutrition facts, 24
Nuts and seeds
about: in salads, 158
Camper's Delight, *115*
Crunchy Fruit Creation, *115*

Oatmeal. *See* Cereal
Olives, 159
Online shopping, 77
Open-Faced Chicken Quesadilla, *98*
Open-Faced Mexican Veggie Burrito, *92*
Orange-Fennel Pasta, *58*
Out-to-Lunch Calorie IQ (by vendor), 118

Pantry
must-haves, 36
purging, 34
Papaya, about, 88
Parties. *See Sweet celebrations references*
Pasta
about: cooking whole-grain, 58; eating out, 174; hall of shame restaurant dishes (by vendor), 174; picking, 85
Chicken and Artichoke Pasta, *98*
Confetti Pasta, *58*
Creamy Mushroom Cavatappi, *175*
Marinara Pasta, *59*
Orange-Fennel Pasta, *58*
Pasta Salad with Chicken and Mixed Veggies, *92*
Pasta with Peas and Onion, *59*
Pasta with Tomatoes and Lemon, *59*
Pasta with Tuna Puttanesca, *79*
Spinach and Tortellini, *91*
Spinach and White Bean Pasta, *91*
Steak Pesto Pasta, *101*
Thai Steak Noodles, *101*
Whole-Wheat Penne Genovese, *177*
PB and B, *115*

PB Pudding, *68*
Peaches and Cream, *68*
Pears
    about, 93
    Poached Pears with Fresh
        Ginger, *179*
Pilates, 202
Pita Spread, *38*
Pizza, 60, 105
Poached Pears with Fresh
    Ginger, *179*
Popcorn calories, 120
Pork. *See* Meat
Portion control. *See* Serving
    sizes
Potatoes
    about: substitute for French
        fries, 44
    Holiday Herb-Roasted
        Potatoes, *218*
    Light Latkes, *226*
    Potato Salad, *236*
    Shepherd's Pie, *67*
Produce. *See also* Fruits;
    Vegetables
    Daily Calorie Targets and, 17
    shopping tips, 88–95
Protein
    Daily Calorie Targets and, 17
    shopping for meat, poultry,
        and seafood, 96–101
    substituting ingredients to
        optimize, 28–29
    what to look for, 23
Provençal Sauce, *63*
Pumpkin Spice Ring, *224*

Quiznos choices, 160

Recipes, list of, 32–33. *See
    also specific recipes or main
    ingredients*
Red-Cooked Chicken with
    Assorted Vegetables, *61*
Red Pepper and Goat Cheese
    Omelet, *41*
Refrigerator/freezer must-
    haves, 35, 37
Restaurants. *See* Eating out
Rice, in Steak Fried Rice, *101*
Roasted Salmon with Squash, *65*

Salad dressings
    healthy (by brand), 95
    light, 159
    swapping full-fat for spray, 49
Salads
    about: beans in, 158; cheese
        in, 159; chicken in, 159;
        eating out (by vendor), 163;
        eggs in, 159; as first course,
        56; fresh veggies/fruit in,
        158; greens in, 158; nuts and
        seeds in, 158; olives in, 159;
        top for lunch, 45; top salad
        bar choices, 158–159
    Chicken and Rice Salad, *45*
    Dijon Bean and Veggie
        Salad, *45*
    Garbanzo Bean Salad, *50*
    Greek Steak Salad, *101*
    Honey Mustard Chicken
        Salad, *45*
    Lime Tuna and Black Bean
        Salad, *45*
    Pasta Salad with Chicken and
        Mixed Veggies, *92*
    Potato Salad, *236*
    Salmon and Black Bean
        Tortilla Salad, *79*
    Spinach Salad with Chicken, *91*
    Sweet and Savory Salmon
        Salad, *45*
    Tuna Salad, *48*
    Tuscan Tuna Salad, *79*
    Waldorf Salad, *98*
Salmon. *See* Fish and seafood
Sandwiches
    about: bread for, 156; brown
        bag lunches, 116; eating
        out, 156–157; 450-calorie
        sandwich, 46–47; Greek
        makeover, 172; healthy
        frozen heat-and-eat (by
        brand), 105; list of healthy
        recipes, 32. *See also specific
        recipes or main ingredients*;
        ordering lean fillings, 156;
        piling on veggies, 156;
        skipping mayo, 156; slimmer,
        to reduce calories, 222
    Caribbean Wrap, *98*
    Greek Chicken Burgers, *173*
    Mediterranean Couscous, *98*
    Open-Faced Chicken
        Quesadilla, *98*
    Open-Faced Mexican Veggie
        Burrito, *92*
    Spinach and Hummus
        Flatbread, *91*
    Steak Fajita Wraps, *101*
    Tuna English Muffins, *79*
    Tuna Salad, *48*
    Tuscan Tuna Salad, *79*
    Waffle Sandwich, *115*
Sandwich spreads, 47, 156
Sauces, spreads and dips
    about: healthy salad
        dressings (by brand), 95;
        sandwich spreads, 47, 156
    Apple-Curry Sauce, *62*
    Black Bean Dip, *50*
    Black Bean Salsa, *63*
    Chinese Ginger Sauce, *63*
    Dijon Sauce, *62*
    Guiltless Guacamole, *167*
    Pita Spread, *38*
    Provençal Sauce, *63*
    Sour Cream and Onion Party
        Dip, *242*
Serving sizes
    downsizing, 30
    parties and, 238, 239
    reading labels, 24, 76
    restaurant portion control,
        144–145
Sesame Shrimp and Asparagus
    Stir-Fry, *169*
Shepherd's Pie, *67*
Shopping (supermarket savvy)
    about: overview of, 73
    for canned and dry goods,
        78–80
    Daily Calorie Targets and, 77
    for dairy, 102–104
    Do It Now, 80, 81, 86
    eating before, 75, 212
    family participation and, 75
    for frozen food, 105–107
    for grains, 84–87
    Learn from the "Losers,"
        95, 100
    Make It a Habit, 83, 90, 103
    for meat, poultry, and
        seafood, 96–101
    online, 77

reading labels, 24, 76
for snacks and drinks (by
  brand), 81–83
sticking to list, 74
Stop the Cart tips, 90, 93,
  99, 104
top 5 tips, 74–76
working the edges, 75
Shrimp. *See* Fish and seafood
Side-dish recipe list, 33
Simple Swaps
  diet soda for soda, 36
  English muffin for bagel, 60
  full-fat for spray salad
    dressing, 49
  orange for orange juice, 34
  skim milk for whole, 54
Sleep, 124
Slow cookers, 61
Smoothies, *115*, 154, *155*
Snacks. *See also* Sweet
  celebrations
  calorie-controlled, stocking, 53
  candy calorie savings, 127
  eating in, 52–55
  exercise and, 198–201
  50-calorie salty, 52
  50-calorie sweet, 52
  healthy convenience options
    (by brand), 81
  healthy crackers
    (by brand), 87
  Learn from the "Losers,"
    55, 71, 95
  100-calorie dairy, 55
  100-calorie fruits/veggies, 54
  100-calorie hearty helpings, 55
  100-calorie savory bites, 55
  100-calorie sweet, 54
  popcorn calories, 120
  shopping for drinks and,
    81–83
  smart, 52–55, 81, 198
  to stash (by brand), 121
  three-day meal plan, 20–21
  tracking wrappers, 214
  traveling and, 131
  vending machine
    know-how, 120
  at work, 111, 112, 120–121
  workouts replacing, 55
Snow Pea Stir-Fry, *92*

Soups
  about: healthy canned or
    boxed, 78; shopping for, 78;
    soup lunch, 116; starting
    meal with, 227
  Black Bean Soup, *51*
  Kidney Bean Chili, *51*
  New England Clam
    Chowder, *66*
Sour Cream and Onion Party
  Dip, *242*
Spicing up meals, 60
Spinach
  about: nutritional value of,
    90; top 5 meal ideas for
    prewashed bagged, 91
  Spinach and Hummus
    Flatbread, *91*
  Spinach and Tortellini, *91*
  Spinach and White Bean
    Pasta, *91*
  Spinach, Cheese, and Bacon
    Omelet, *41*
  Spinach Salad with Chicken, *91*
  Spinach Scramble, *91*
Squash (butternut), about, 89
Standing for slimming, 205
Steak. *See* Meat
Strawberries. *See* Berries
Strength training, 192–197
Stress management, 126, 216
Stuffing, Vegetable-Herb, *223*
Substituting ingredients, 28–29
Subway choices, 160
Sugar alternatives, 80
Sugar, reducing, 80
Supermarket savvy. *See*
  Shopping (supermarket savvy)
Sushi mix up (by type), 162
Sweet and Salty, *115*
Sweet and Savory Salmon
  Salad, *45*
Sweet celebrations
  about: overview of, 209
  activities for burning calories
    and, 227, 228. *See also*
    Exercise
  alcoholic beverage calories
    and, 244–245
  being at peace with cravings,
    213
  being waiter/waitress at, 228

better BBQ savings, 235
buffet behaviors and, 213
cake consumption
  and, 239, *241*
calorie cheat sheet, 243
carrying mint sprig
  during, 220
Daily Calorie Targets
  and, 212
Do It Now, 214, 220, 227, 243
dropping all-or-nothing
  attitude for, 213
Easter sweets and eggs, 232
exercise and, 211
guilt-free grilling and, 234
Halloween help, 215, 217
hors d'oeuvres calories
  and, 239
keeping your hands
  occupied at, 231
leftovers and, 222
Make It a Habit, 217, 222,
  227, 228, 231, 236, 240
not cleaning your plate
  at, 240
party-proofing diet for,
  238, 240
passing out candy at, 217
PDA party help, 225
picky eating at, 210
portion control guidelines
  for, 238, 239
preparing for, 210
seasonal stress and, 216
simple substitutions for, 219
slimmer sandwiches for, 222
starving yourself before, 239
terrifying treats
  (by brand), 214
top 5 tips, 210–213
Valentine's Day quiz, 231
warm weather gatherings,
  234–237
weighing yourself before and
  after, 227
Sweet celebrations (recipes)
  about: reducing calories
    with, 219; reducing side-
    dish calories, 220
  Angel Food Cake, *241*
  Better Banana Pudding, *237*

Holiday Herb-Roasted
Potatoes, *218*
Hot Cocoa Mix, *230*
Lean Green Bean
Casserole, *221*
Light and Creamy
Eggnog, *229*
Lighter Brownies, *233*
Light Latkes, *226*
Potato Salad, *236*
Pumpkin Spice Ring, *224*
Sour Cream and Onion Party
Dip, *242*
Vegetable-Herb Stuffing, *223*
Sweet potatoes, about, 89

Tai Chi, 203
Thai Steak Noodles, *101*
Thirst, mistaking for hunger, 120
Three-day meal plan, 20–21
Tofu, 99
Traveling, 130–133
Tuna. *See* Fish and seafood
Turkey
about: healthy convenience
options (by brand), 96;
slimming sandwiches, 222
Turkey Fajitas, *171*

Valentine's Day quiz, 231
Vegetable-Herb Stuffing, *223*
Vegetables. *See also specific
vegetables*
as first course, 56
frozen, nutrition of, 93
frozen, top 5 meal ideas for, 92
healthiest, characteristics
of, 88
healthy convenience options
(by brand), 94
juice benefits, 64
not eating enough, 94
100-calorie snacks, 54
preprepped, 90–91
in salads. *See* Salads
shopping for fruits and,
88–95
Vegetarian, eating once weekly, 44

Waffle Sandwich, *115*
Waldorf Salad, *98*
Walking, 122, 186–191, 207, 216

Water, drinking, 128, 236
Watermelon, about, 88
Water workouts, 203
Weight loss. *See also* Calories
believing in, 22
calcium-rich diets and, 103
calories per pound, 10
changing/maintaining
habits, 25
creating calorie deficit for, 10
diets and, 8
discounting little things, 126
the Drop 5 way, 11
dropping all-or-nothing
attitude, 213
eating in and. *See* Eating in
eating out and. *See* Eating out
getting facts about foods
and, 23
at healthy pace, 10
losing more than five pounds, 9
mistaking thirst for hunger
and, 120
for money, 124
optimizing calories, 22–23
physical activity and, 25. *See
also* Exercise; Fitness
science of, 10
spot-reducing myth, 197
staying on track at work,
124–129
strategies, 22–25
substituting ingredients and,
28–29
whittling your middle, 196
Western-Style Omelet, *41*
Whole-Wheat Penne
Genovese, *177*
Workplace
about: overview of, 110
breakfasts and, 114–115
breaking bad behaviors at, 125
brown bag lunches for,
110–111, 116
buddying up at, 110
candy dish facts and calorie
savings and, 127
curbing all-day nibbling at, 122
desktop dining at, 117
Do It Now, 113, 117, 125, 128,
129, 130
drinking water at, 128

frequent breaks at, 129
getting healthy choices in
cafeteria, 117
Learn from the "Losers,"
123, 129
lunches and munchies,
116–121
Make It a Habit, 117, 122,
128, 131
mixing up food routine at, 111
not eating what you don't
want at, 117
planning when/where to
eat at, 113
snacks at, 111, 112, 120–121
staying on track at, 124–129
top 5 how-tos for, 110–112
traveling and working on the
road, 130–133
vending machine know-how
for, 120
weight-loss incentives
from, 124
working out at, 112, 122–123,
128, 130

Yoga, 126, 203
Yogurt, healthy (by brand), 103

PHOTOGRAPHY CREDITS

Courtesy of Diana Abdel-Rahman: 162 (Abdel-Rahman "before")

Ge Fotostock: Jeremy Woodhouse: 206

Courtesy of Annie's: 95 (salad dressing)

James Baigrie: 219, 229, 235 & 236 (light potato salad)

Be heard photography: 69, 101

Courtesy of Sarah Bell: 205 (Bell "before")

Courtesy of Bumblebee Tuna: 100 (tuna)

Courtesy of Burger King: 163

Alex Cao: 53

Courtesy of Jessica Chicas: 71 (Chicas "before")

Con Poulous: 67, 104 (egg)

Corbis Images: Patrick Lane/Somos: 4 (cereal); Beau Lark: 4 (baking); Brooke Fasani: Roulier/Turiot/PhotoCuisine: 168, 202; David Selman, 211 (cake)

Courtesy of Denny's: 149 (Lumberjack Slam)

Tara Donne: 32 & 167 (guacamole); 33 & 70 (cookies); 33 & 57 (meatloaf); 59, 61 (chicken); 62 (chicken); 167, 173 (burger)

Courtesy of Dove Chocolate: 107 (ice cream bar)

Courtesy Dunkin' Donuts: 147, 153 (Coolatta)

Denise Foley: 99

Courtesy of Kim Francis: 191 (Francis "before")

Connor Gleason: 86 (oatmeal); 102, 107 (Häagen-Dazs, Edy's, Weight Watchers, Ben & Jerry's, Breyers); 118, 141, 146 (protein plate); 150 (parfait & granola); 151, 153 (Starbucks, Burger King, McCafe, Wendy's); 201 (Whopper); 217 (McDonnald's); 225 (Edy's)

Courtesy of Jan Haapala: 55

Gregor Halenda: 37 (frozen dinners)

Getty Images: amana productions inc: 134; Jack Andersen: 236 (seltzer); Armstrong Studios: 179; Jan Baumann/STOCK 4B: 211 (sandwiches); Leigh Beisch: 172, 220 (potatoes); Annabelle Breakey: 224; Burke/Triolo Productions: 207; Renee Comet: 62 (potato); George Doyle: 27 (woman), 156; Sam Edwards: 112; Britt Erianson: 196 (lifting weights); Richard Eskite: 96 (stir fry); Foodcollection: 21 (soup), 47 (pesto); Fuse/Jupiter Images: 212; Jules Frazier: 119 (sandwich); Gentl and Hyers: 99 (tofu); Aaron Graubart and Anderson Ross: 80 (magnifying glass); JGI/Jamie Grill: 231 (friends); Brian Hagiwara: 243 (shrimp); Pando Hall: 103 (woman); GK Hart/Vikki Hart: 103 (cow); Philip Lee Harvey: 123 (couple); Paula Hible: 115; Hill Street Studios: 76 (woman); Image Source: 240 (party); Imagewerks: 190 (woman); James and James: 52; Jeff Kauck: 40 (sour cream); John Kelly: 187 (hiking); Dorling Kindersley: 159 (cheese), 243 (cheese straws); Peter LaMastro: 188; Darryl Leniuk: 180; Joseph De Leo: 173 (fries); Martine Mouchy: 128; Neo Vision: 108; Amy Neunsinger: 234 (grilling); Judd Pilossof: 40 (omelet); Tim Platt: 16; Steven Puetzer: 222 (leftovers); David Prince: 235 (regular potato salad); Rubberball: 205 (standing woman); Jim Scherer: 49 (sandwich); Smneedham: 107 (ice cream bar), 201 (fries); David De Stefano: 199 (cookie); Southern Stock: 34 (orange juice); Stockbyte: 4 & 187 (woman walking), 71 (donut), 89 (broccoli), 139 (woman); Tetra Images: 11; Martina Urban: 49 (rice); Westend61: 25

Courtesy of Jan Haapala: 55 (Haapala "before")

iStock: 4kodia: 39 (sausage); Tim Abramowitz : 127; Monika Adamczyk: 21 & 155 (smoothie); ALEAIMAGE: 47 (ketchup); AlexStar: 88 (kiwi); Carlos Alvarez: 189 (bicycle); Andresr: 4 & 181 (woman stretching); Andyd: 89 (whole squash); Andrey Artykov: 183 (cycling); aspenrock: 44 (burger); Lonni Aylett: 125 (plate); Leslie Banks: 154 (sausage); Barbro Bergfeldt: 45, 175 (salad); Eddie Berman: 210 (drink); Chris Bernard: 197; Joe Biafore: 158 (blueberries); Mariya Bibikova: 159 (oil); Oliver Blondeau: 34 & 50 (orange), 109 (breakfast); Natasha Bo: 97 (ribs); Felix Brandl: 80 (sugar); Hilary Brodey: 56 (edamame), 83; Claire Broomfield: 137; Daniel R. Burch: 144 (dice); John Burwell: 20 & 154 (oatmeal); Aleksey Butov: 54 (whole milk); Cedric Carter: 214 (peanut butter cups); Kin Shing Chan: 14; Norman Chan: 91; Jill Chen: 46, 110 (sandwich); Junghee Choi: 59 (salmon); Kelly Cline: 21 (sandwich), 28 (fish), 76 (broccolini), 114 (parfait), 210 (cheese), 144 (pasta); creacart: 144 (chocolate); christopher Conrad: 268; Agnes Csondor: 213; Shane Cummins: 125 (carrots); Lachlan Currie: 20 (mango); Robert Dant: 145 (pancake); Dennis DeSilva: 162 (edamame); Sergei Didok: 245 (wine); Diane Diederich: 209 (cake); DNY59: 89 (brussels sprouts), 227 (soup), 228 (milk); Philip Dyer: 190 (tape measure); Ekspansio: 158 (tomato); Rebecca Ellis: 244 (bloody mary); Chris Elwell: 64 (mock-pie); Donald Erickson: 41 (melon), 42 (oatmeal), 51 (chips), 59 (broccoli), 63 (couscous), 144 (roll); E_Y_E: 159 (egg);

felinda: 88 (papaya); Greg Ferguson: 240 (pie); Laura Fischer: 145 (compact); Floortje: 98, 162 (sushi); FotografiaBasica: 56 (bulgur), 145 (oil); david franklin: 110 (bag); FreezeFrameStudio: 84; Stephanie Frey: 239 (pigs in a blanket); Liv Friis-Larsen: 154 (yogurt); Jill Fromer: 198 (energy bar), 231 (heart), 234 (flag); futureimage: 245 (mimosa); Peter Garbet: 42 (café au lait); Justine Gecewicz: 93 (shortcake); Natalya Gerasimova: 86 (raspberries); gerenme: 35 (refrigerator), 228 (tray); Hedda Gjerpen: 204 (horseback); Spencer Gordon: 126; Joe Gough: 174; Samantha Grandy: 149 (pancakes); Michael Gray: 154 (egg); Bill Grove: 88 (watermelon); Eva Gruendemann: 164 (rice & veggies); Ermin Gutenberger: 34 & 243 (potato chips), 158 (walnuts); HannamariaH: 93 (light shortcake); Sitan Magnus Hatling: 120 (water); haveseen: 244 (mojito); Mostafa Hefni: 154 (biscuit); Bjorn Heller: 200 (beer); Rubén Hidalgo: 74 (shopping list); Joshua Hodge Photography: 29; Danny Hooks: 170 (margarita); Carey Hope: 18; Gord Horne: 198 (fruit & nuts); Václav Hroch: 10 & 183 (woman); ingmarsan: 158 (lettuce); intst: 41 & 88 (grapefruit); Rafa Irusta: 86 (cereal); ivanastar: 232 (eggs); Gabor Izso: 51 (blackberries), 155 (strawberries); James and James: 52 (ice pop); Jesus Jauregui: 125 (gum); Matt Jeacock: 238 (hats); Kristen Johansen: 203; Paul Johnson: 12 (cola); jsemeniuk: 216; Juanmonino: 58 (shrimp), 60 (muffin), 144 (salmon); Ju-Lee: 154 (fruit cup), 214 (jack-o-lantern); edis jurcys: 243 (sausage); Jack Kelly: 27 (potatoes); kivoart: 78 (soup); Adam Korzekwa: 43 (berries); Maya Kovacheva: 89 (yam); Michael Krinke: 59 & 159 (chicken); Gethin Lane: 92; Uyen Le: 41 (raspberries), 66 (salad); Tomaz Levstek: 130 (door); Joshua Lewis: 217 (lollipops); lillisphotograph: 136 (menu); Daniel Loiselle: 57 (potato); Cat London: 226 (dreidles); Olga Lyubkina: 145 (bagel); Robyn Mackenzie: 38, 62 (rice), 170 (fajita); ma-k: 64 (tomato juice), 200 (tea); Erkki Makkonen: 87 (crispbread); travis manley: 34 (soda); Maridav: 185; John A Meents: 111; Michael_at_isp: 35 (cheese); Daniel Mitchell: 245 (rum & Diet Coke); monica-photo: 165; Morgan Lane Studios: 94 (woman shopping), 144 (mouse); Ann Murie: 135 (fork); naphtalina: 164 (buffet); Neustockimages: 9, 26; Stacey Newman: 12 (pizza), 34 (bread); Julia Nichols: 61 (crock pot); Alexander Novikov: 189 (aerobics); Leonid Nyshko: 145 (nuts & fruit); Sandra O'Claire: 239 (cupcake); Monika Olszewska: 244 (gin & tonic); pagadesign: 124; Marina Parshina: 97 (tenderloin); Lauri Patterson: 143; Robert Payne: 12 & 245 (beer); Miljan Petrovic: 93 (green beans); rico Ploeg: 215 (apple pie); Joe Potato: 36 (sauce); Anton Prado: 144 (glass); Paul Prescott: 74 (shopping cart); Pumba 1: 75; ranplett: 88 (strawberry); Punchstock: 182; Pali Rao: 139 (menu); RedHelga: 159 (olives); Paul Rosado: 145 (thumb); Neil Redmond: 64 (pot pie); Dirk Rietsche: 44 (fries); Ashok Rodrigues: 231 (cordial); Jan Rysavy: 227 (holly); Elena Schweitzer: 89 (cut squash), 145 (butter); Richard Scherzinger: 35 (yogurt); Angelika Schwarz: 246; Elzbieta Sekowska: 63 (noodles); Branislav Senic: 4 (salmon); sf_foodphoto: 35 (hummus), 136 (salmon); Harris Shiffman: 60 (bagel); Maksim Shmeljov: 184; Victoria Short: 164 (fried rice); ShyMan: 106 (sorbet); Suzannah Skelton: 89 (kale), 153 & 154 (bacon), 162 (california roll); Jerome Skiba: 85 (pasta); Brigitte Smith: 114 (apple & cheese); Danny Smyth: 49 & 144 (salad dressing); james steidl: 73 (groceries); spaxiax: 199 (chips); Serghei Starus: 204 (mitt & ball); Stephen Stiling: 58 (spinach); subjug: 40 (toast); Mark Swallow: 5 (basket); Todd Taulman: 245 (martini); Kevin Thomas: 54 (skim milk); Jason Stitt: 181 (dumbell); Willie B. Thomas: 135 (chefs); Alasdair Thomson: 57 (asparagus), 158 (chick peas); thumb: 130 (water), 144 (ball), 198 (juice); Stefanie Timmermann: 131 (trail mix); Alberto Tirado: 8; Sawayasu Tsuji: 52 & 63 (avocado); Dean Turner: 12 (donut), 25 (apple); Jan Tyler: 230 (candy canes); Simone van den Berg: 196 (kickboxing); Jacob VanHouten: 28 (spatula); Liz Van Steenburgh: 209 (party blowers); Craig Veltri: 217 (candy apple); Marek Walica: 88 (half-grapefruit); Josh Webb: 5 (woman cooking); webphotographeer: 208; Terry Wilson: 204 (jump rope); camilla wisbauer: 55 & 243 (Goldfish crackers); Yasonya: 39 (grapefruit); Nicole S. Young: 99 (salmon); Tomasz Zachariasz: 109 (briefcase); Dusan Zidar: 20 & 68 (ice cream); Kenneth C. Zirkel: 5 & 116 (lunch); Maria Zoroyan: 58 (pasta)

Courtesy of KFC: 140, 161
Courtesy of Josie Latimer: 207 (Latimer "before")
Courtesy of Donna Lennart: 129 (Lennart "before")
David Lewis Taylor: 132—133
Rita Maas: 169, 218
Kate Mathis: 4 & 66 (clam chowder); 32 & 48

(sandwich); 43 (french toast); 33 & 226 (latkes); 39 (muffins); 48, 65, 171, 221, 223, 226, 233; 240 (Apple Delight); 242

Hilmar Meyer-Bosse: 95 (Spirou "after"), 35 (Sanchez "after"), 123 (Skiles "after"), 129 (Lennart "after"), 191 (Francis "after"), 205 (Bell "after"), 207 (Latimer "after")

Courtesy of Olive Garden: 166

Courtesy of Panera: 157

Punchstock: Photodisc: 227 (woman with snowman)

Courtesy of Sara Lee: 87 (bread)

Courtesy of Heather Sanchez: 35 (Sanchez "before")

Kate Sears: 175 (cavatappi), 177

Courtesy of Lisa Skiles: 123 (Skiles "before")

Courtesy of Chris Spirou: 95 (Spirou "before")

Stockfood: Buchanan Studios Inc: 237; Foodcollection: 13 (french fries)

Courtesy of Stonyfield: 103 (yogurt)

Ann Stratton: 44 (baked fries)

Studio D: 17 (grapes), 54; 106 (ice cream bar); Jesus Ayala: 50 (beans); Chris Eckert: 35 (egg), 55 (soup), 120 (Campbell's, Mott's, South Beach, Earthbound, Sun Chips, Blue Bunny, Yoplait, Cracker Barrel, Fudgsicle, Barbara's), 145 (egg, DVD); Philip Friedman: 13 (cookies), 17 (rice, almonds), 23, 36 (mustard), 49 (salad spray), 50 (pita), 51 (cheese), 52 (Ak-mak), 54 (brownies), 55 (cheese, Haapala "after"), 71 (Chicas "after"), 78 (can), 79, 81, 82, 85 (rice), 93 (pear), 94 (beets), 96 (chicken), 100 (salmon), 104 (egg whites), 105, 106, 107 & 108 (Fudgsicles, Whole Treat bars), 120 (popcorn), 121 (purse); 129 (prunes, pedometer), 130 (pretzels), 144 (iphone), 146 (oatmeal), 148, 150 (Egg McFuffin), 152 (muffins, scone), 160, 178, 191 (pedometer), 200 (smoothie), 215 (M & M's), 217 (book), 232 (Peeps & Jellybeans, Cadbury, Whoppers), 241, 243 (popcorn, pretzels, peanuts); Karl Juengel: 60 (pizza slices), 145 (scrabble tile); J Muckle: 36 (Coke), 90, 131 (Blackberry), 153 (McDonald's), 222 (turkey sandwiches); Lara Robby: 36 (Diet Coke), 54 (strawberries), 176, 198 (banana), 215 (Hershey's bar, Tootsie Roll, Skittles, Smarties, Rolos, Butterfinger, Hershey's Kisses, Charms, Dum Dums), 225 (pecan pie), 230 (Starbucks), 231 (strawberry); David Turner: 162 (Abdel-Rahman "after"); Jeffrey Westbrook: 220 (mint)

Courtesy of Taco Bell: 119 (nachos, tacos)

Jason Todd: 192–195

Mark Thomas: 238 (buffet)

Veer: Alloy Photography: 4 (wine glasses), 117; Corbis Photography: 72; Fancy Photography: 73 (woman)

Anna Williams: 230 (cocoa)

Front cover: Courtesy of Dunkin' Donuts (egg sandwich); iStock: Floortje (chicken); Dean Turner (doughnut); Dirk Rietschel (fries); Ann Stratton (baked fries); Mark Swallow (shopping basket)

Front flap: Getty Images: Tim Platt (woman in jeans); iStock: Kelly Cline (parfait)

Spine: iStock: paul prescott

Back cover: iStock: Kelly Cline: 46 (sandwich); Studio D: Karl Juengel (pizza)

Back flap: Tara Donne (cookies)

METRIC EQUIVALENT CHARTS

THE RECIPES IN THIS BOOK use the standard United States method for measuring liquid and dry or solid ingredients (teaspoons, tablespoons, and cups). The information on this chart is provided to help cooks outside the U.S. successfully use these recipes. All equivalents are approximate.

METRIC EQUIVALENTS FOR DIFFERENT TYPES OF INGREDIENTS

A standard cup measure of a dry or solid ingredient will vary in weight depending on the type of ingredient. A standard cup of liquid is the same volume for any type of liquid. Use the following chart when converting standard cup measures to grams (weight) or milliliters (volume).

Standard Cup	Fine Powder (e.g. flour)	Grain (e.g. rice)	Granular (e.g. sugar)	Liquid Solids (e.g. butter)	Liquid (e.g. milk)
1	140 g	150 g	190 g	200 g	240 ml
¾	105 g	113 g	143 g	150 g	180 ml
⅔	93 g	100 g	125 g	133 g	160 ml
½	70 g	75 g	95 g	100 g	120 ml
⅓	47 g	50 g	63 g	67 g	80 ml
¼	35 g	38 g	48 g	50 g	60 ml
⅛	18 g	19 g	24 g	25 g	30 ml

USEFUL EQUIVALENTS FOR LIQUID INGREDIENTS BY VOLUME

¼ tsp	=					1 ml
½ tsp	=					2 ml
1 tsp	=					5 ml
3 tsp	=	1 tbls =		½ fl oz	=	15 ml
		2 tbls =	⅛ cup =	1 fl oz	=	30 ml
		4 tbls =	¼ cup =	2 fl oz	=	60 ml
		5⅓ tbls =	⅓ cup =	3 fl oz	=	80 ml
		8 tbls =	½ cup =	4 fl oz	=	120 ml
		10⅔ tbls =	⅔ cup =	5 fl oz	=	160 ml
		12 tbls =	¾ cup =	6 fl oz	=	180 ml
		16 tbls =	1 cup =	8 fl oz	=	240 ml
		1 pt =	2 cups =	16 fl oz	=	480 ml
		1 qt =	4 cups =	32 fl oz	=	960 ml
				33 fl oz	=	1000 ml = 1 L

USEFUL EQUIVALENTS FOR DRY INGREDIENTS BY WEIGHT

(To convert ounces to grams, multiply the number of ounces by 30.)

1 oz	=	¹⁄₁₆ lb	=	30 g
2 oz	=	¼ lb	=	120 g
4 oz	=	½ lb	=	240 g
8 oz	=	¾ lb	=	360 g
16 oz	=	1 lb	=	480 g

USEFUL EQUIVALENTS FOR COOKING/OVEN TEMPERATURES

	Fahrenheit	Celsius	Gas Mark
Freeze Water	32° F	0° C	
Room Temperature	68° F	20° C	
Boil Water	212° F	100° C	
Bake	325° F	160° C	3
	350° F	180° C	4
	375° F	190° C	5
	400° F	200° C	6
	425° F	220° C	7
	450° F	230° C	8
Broil			Grill

USEFUL EQUIVALENTS FOR LENGTH

(To convert inches to centimeters, multiply the number of inches by 2.5.)

1 in	=			2.5 cm		
6 in	=	½ ft	=	15 cm		
12 in	=	1 ft	=	30 cm		
36 in	=	3 ft	= 1 yd =	90 cm		
40 in	=			100 cm	=	1 m

THE GOOD HOUSEKEEPING TRIPLE-TEST PROMISE

At *Good Housekeeping*, we want to make sure that every recipe we print works in any oven, with any brand of ingredient, no matter what. That's why, in our test kitchens at the GOOD HOUSEKEEPING RESEARCH INSTITUTE, we go all out: We test each recipe at least three times—and, often, several more times after that. When a recipe is first developed, one member of our team prepares the dish and we judge it on these criteria: It must be DELICIOUS, FAMILY-FRIENDLY, HEALTHY, and EASY TO MAKE.

1   The recipe is then tested several more times to fine-tune the flavor and ease of preparation, always by the same team member, using the same equipment.

2   Next, another team member follows the recipe as written, VARYING THE BRANDS OF INGREDIENTS and KINDS OF EQUIPMENT. Even the types of stoves we use are changed.

3   A third team member repeats the whole process USING YET ANOTHER SET OF EQUIPMENT and ALTERNATIVE INGREDIENTS.

BY THE TIME THE RECIPES APPEAR ON THESE PAGES, THEY ARE GUARANTEED TO WORK IN ANY KITCHEN, INCLUDING YOURS. WE PROMISE.

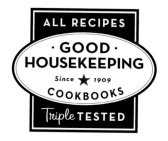

GOOD HOUSEKEEPING

Rosemary Ellis, *Editor in Chief*

Jennifer L. Cook, *Executive Editor*

Courtney Murphy, *Design Director*

Toni Gerber Hope, *Health Director*

Sara Lyle, *Lifestyle Editor*

Trent Johnson, *Art Director*

Susan Westmoreland, *Food Director,*
Good Housekeeping Research Institute

Samantha B. Cassetty, MS, RD, *Nutrition Director,*
Good Housekeeping Research Institute

With thanks to Kate Winne, RD; Beth Sumrell Ehrensberger, MPH, RD; and Tamara Goldis, RD.

Book design by Nancy Leonard

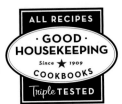

ALL RECIPES
·GOOD·
HOUSEKEEPING
Since ★ 1909
COOKBOOKS
Triple TESTED

Published by Hearst Books
A division of Sterling Publishing Co., Inc.
387 Park Avenue South, New York, NY 10016

Good Housekeeping is a registered trademark of Hearst Communications, Inc.
www.goodhousekeeping.com

For information about custom editions, special sales, premium and corporate purchases, please contact Sterling Special Sales Department at 800-805-5489 or specialsales@sterlingpublishing.com.

Distributed in Canada by Sterling Publishing
c/o Canadian Manda Group, 165 Dufferin Street
Toronto, Ontario, Canada M6K 3H6

Distributed in Australia by Capricorn Link
(Australia) Pty. Ltd.
P.O. Box 704, Windsor, NSW 2756 Australia

Printed in the USA

Sterling ISBN 978-1-58816-786-6

Library of Congress Cataloging-in-Publication Data
Jones, Heather K.
  Good housekeeping drop 5 lbs : the small changes, big results diet/
Heather K. Jones ;
Rosemary Ellis, editor-in-chief, Good housekeeping.
    p. cm.
  Includes index.
  ISBN 978-1-58816-786-6
1. Weight loss. 2. Energy metabolism. 3. Reducing diet. 4.
Alternative lifestyles. I. Good housekeeping. II. Title. III. Title: Good housekeeping drop five pounds.
  RM222.2.J6168 2010
  613.2'5--dc22
        2010018434